The Eye in General Practice

C. R. S. Jackson
MA DM (Oxon) DOMS FRCS (Edin.)
Formerly Consultant Ophthalmic Surgeon, Royal
Infirmary, Edinburgh and Clinical Tutor in
Ophthalmology, University of Oxford

R. D. Finlay
MA BM BCh (Oxon) FRCS FRCS (Edin.) DO
Consultant Ophthalmic Surgeon, Royal United
Hospital, Bath and formerly Postgraduate
Clinical Tutor, Bath

EIGHTH EDITION

CHURCHILL LIVINGSTONE
EDINBURGH LONDON MELBOURNE AND NEW YORK 1985

CHURCHILL LIVINGSTONE
Medical Division of Longman Group UK Limited

Distributed in the United States of America by
Churchill Livingstone Inc., 1560 Broadway, New York,
N.Y. 10036, and by associated companies, branches and
representatives throughout the world.

First edition 1957
Second edition 1960
Third edition 1964
Fourth edition 1967
Fifth edition 1969
Sixth edition 1972
Seventh edition 1975
Eighth edition 1985
  Reprinted 1988

ISBN 0 443 03213 0

British Library Cataloguing in Publication Data
Jackson, C.R.S.
    The eye in general practice. — 8th ed.
    1. Eye — Diseases and defects
    I. Title   II. Finlay, R.D.
    617.7   RE46

Library of Congress Cataloging in Publication Data
Jackson, C.R.S. (Charles Robert Sweeting)
    The eye in general practice.
    Includes index.
    1. Ocular manifestations of general diseases.
    I. Finlay, R.D.   II. Title. [DNLM: 1. Eye
Diseases. 2. Eye Manifestations. WW 100 J12e]
    RE65.J34   1985   617.7   84–17031

Produced by Longman Group (FE) Ltd
Printed in Hong Kong

Preface

General practitioners still bemoan their ignorance of ophthalmology, a subject for which there is little time in the undergraduate medical curriculum and scarcely more in the average general practitioner's vocational training programme.

Ophthalmology is a rapidly expanding field, and whilst some changes have little impact on general practice, others are of great importance. New drugs appear all the time, and the general practitioner must have some knowledge of the drugs he is asked to prescribe. Surgical techniques change — intra-ocular lenses, for example, are in everyday use and patients may expect guidance from the general practitioner.

Perhaps the innovation of greatest consequence, and one to which some attention has been given in this edition, is the general availability of argon laser treatment to diabetics with retinopathy. Sadly, the other vascular complications continue unchecked, but much can be done to reduce the diabetic's chance of becoming blind. The role of the general practitioner in screening patients for referral is now crucial. A few years ago, when little could be done, it was less important. Some means must be found in every practice to fulfil this need; not all doctors will approach the problem in the same way.

Ten years have passed since the last edition of *The Eye in General Practice*. The present edition, now under joint authorship, has been completely rewritten. The authors are very much aware of a change in the style expected in medical books in an age when information is abundant and time scarce. The problem-oriented layout has much to commend it, compared with the more conventional, anatomically arranged format. However it is difficult to apply this approach rigorously to eye disorders, so in the present edition a compromise is attempted. Chapter 2 is set out as an analysis of common problems presenting to the general practitioner and references are given to the subsequent chapters, which are arranged on an anatomical basis.

It is the authors' hope that the reader will find in this book a useful bridge between general practice and ophthalmology.

1985

C. R. S. J.
R. D. F.

Acknowledgments

The authors are indebted to many colleagues for advice, particularly Messrs J. D. Griffiths and D. E. P. Jones, and Drs J. Heber, P. G. Mann and J. P. D. Reckless, all of Bath. They are also deeply grateful to colleagues who have kindly provided illustrations: Dr T. Barrie of Glasgow, Dr J. Cairns of Melbourne, Professor S. Darougar of London, Professor D. L. Easty and Mr C. Dean Hart of Bristol, Mr J. Kanski of Windsor, Mr R. S. Mahto of Bath, Mr G. J. Romanes of Dorchester, Dr N. L. Stokoe of Edinburgh and Dr S. Shakir and the radiologists at Bath.

Information about visual standards was kindly provided by Dr H. M. Adams, General Council of British Shipping; Dr W. D. Anderson, British Rail, Bristol; Miss J. M. Gendall, Social Services Department, Bath; Brigadier W. G. Kilpatrick RAMC; Surgeon Commander C. W. Millar RN.; Dr F. S. Preston, British Airways; and Dr J. Taylor, Department of Transport.

For the medical photographers at the Royal United Hospital, Bath, Mrs Gina Machin and Mrs Sally Jenner, nothing appears to have been too much trouble. Most of all, the authors wish to thank RDF's secretary, Mrs R. Barry.

Contents

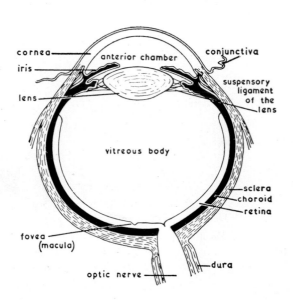

cornea—
iris—
lens—

anterior chamber
conjunctiva
suspensory
ligament
of the
lens

vitreous body

sclera
choroid
retina

fovea
(macula)

dura

optic nerve—

1

History and examination

Ophthalmology is often regarded as a mysterious subject but, as between 1 and 2% of patients attending general practitioners surgeries do so on account of symptoms related to their eyes, some attempt must be made to help in unravelling the various problems.

The eye patient may present with pain, redness, watering, alteration in appearance, impaired or double vision. It must not be forgotten that some with disease of the eye or visual pathway have no complaint.

It is important to note a *history* of previous similar episodes, of any systemic illness, of any eye disease in the family, and the way in which symptoms first present. In particular, bilaterality or otherwise is important. A complaint of sudden visual loss may represent sudden appreciation of a longstanding defect — as, for example, on happening to close or cover the 'good' eye.

The possibility of injury must not be overlooked — especially industrial injury through hammering, drilling, and so on. The nature and distribution of pain may be important. The 'scratchy' pain of a superficial foreign body is quite distinct from the pain of deeper eye disease, which is often referred to brow or cheek, through the branches of the trigeminal nerve.

Equipment

An adequate initial examination of the eye can be made with simple apparatus. The following are minimum requirements:

1. Torch — pen type. Held between finger and thumb, the disengaged fingers resting on the patient's face and, if necessary, helping to keep the eye open (Fig. 1).

2. Magnifier, or loupe ($\times$ 8). For maximum field of view it must be held close to the examiner's eye, while the fingers rest on the patient's face, to maintain focus of the lens.

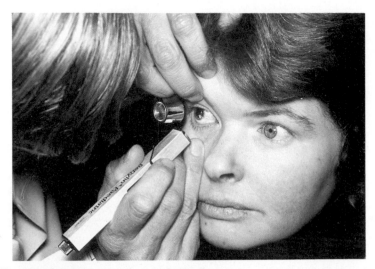

Fig. 1 Examination with torch and loupe

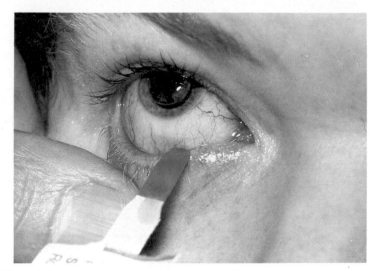

Fig. 2 Staining with fluorescein

3. Fluorescein-impregnated paper strips (Fluorets) moistened by soaking in the tears in the lower part of the conjunctiva (Fig. 2). (NB Never use fluorescein in bottles — danger of contamination, especially by Pseudomonas.) An alternative to fluorescein is rose bengal. Any corneal epithelial defect will pick up the stain; green (fluorescein), or red (rose bengal).

4. Quick-acting, short-lasting mydriatic, to dilate the pupil if need be. Useful drugs are homatropine 2%, cyclopentolate 0.5 or 1.0% (Mydrilate), and tropicamide 0.5 or 1.0%. These are available in disposable, single-dose containers (Minims — SNP). Atropine should be avoided, its effects being unnecessarily powerful and prolonged.

After the examination, a drop of pilocarpine 2% counteracts the effect of the mydriatic. (Mydriasis = dilation of the pupils. Miosis = pupillary constriction.)

5. Ophthalmoscope. Several GP models are available — more useful if the battery is fresh and the bulb not blackened with age. A darkened room makes examination easier: at least, the patient should have his back to the light.

Methods

The first thing to do — and easily overlooked — is to test the vision in each eye separately, with glasses if worn, for both distance and near. (Some patients put on their reading glasses when invited to 'read' the distance test type!) Make sure that the eye not under test is adequately covered. Children, especially, are liable to 'peek'.

The Snellen line labelled '6' (Fig. 3) can be read by the normal eye at 6 metres — hence 6/6. Diminishing ability is represented by 6/9, 6/12, and so on. A test card for near vision is useful, but a newspaper or telephone book will serve.

For young children, and those who cannot read, some kind of illiterate test is needed. Letter matching tests such as the Sheridan-Gardiner (Fig. 4) or Stycar are the most frequently used. The child identifies a letter at 3 or 6 metres and matches it with one of a number of letters on a card held in his hand. Most children of 3 years or older can manage this test, (see p. 109).

Alternatively there is the 'E' test. Capital 'E's corresponding to the Snellen letters and turned in various directions are shown to the child, who responds by indicating the direction in which the legs of the 'E' are pointing.

Visual fields

The test of visual acuity takes account only of the central vision. For completeness, a test of peripheral vision may be made by sitting in front of the patient and comparing the extent of his peripheral vision with one's own, examining the eyes separately (Fig. 5).

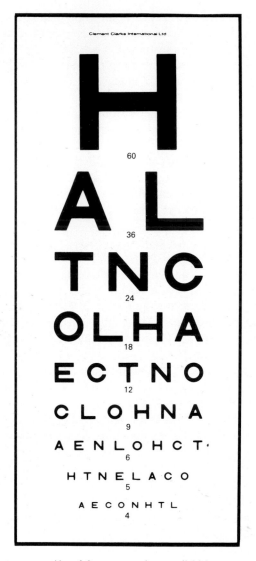

Fig. 3 Snellen test type (6 and 3 metre versions available)

At least, the ability to detect the movement of a hand in each of the four quadrants should be checked. This visual field test may reveal hemianopia from damage to the visual pathways, or field loss from glaucoma, both of which may exist in the presence of normal visual acuity, the patient being unaware of the defect.

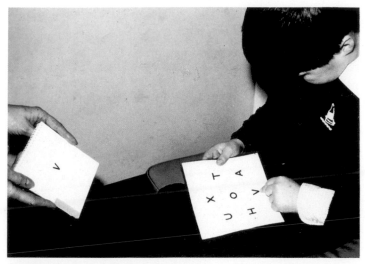

Fig. 4 Sheridan Gardiner test

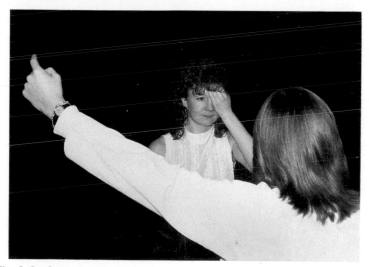

Fig. 5 Confrontation test for visual field

A homonymous defect is most readily demonstrated by the examiner facing the patient and moving both hands (Fig. 6). Failure to see either hand indicates hemianopia: the defect is confirmed by moving the unseen hand across the midline, whereupon the patient is able to see both. This simple test should be repeated in the upper and lower quadrants.

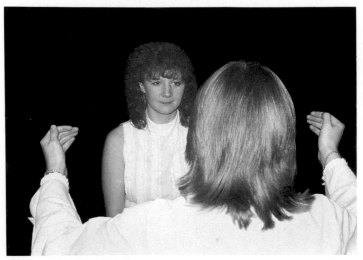

Fig. 6 Test for hemianopia

Eyelids

Symmetry on the two sides is to be expected. Drooping or over-elevation of the upper lid may point to ptosis or lid retraction, perhaps from palsy of the oculomotor nerve or from thyrotoxicosis.

The condition of the skin around the eye is examined, as is the normal position of the eyelashes. Inflammation of the lid margin may be noted, or swellings in the lid substance.

The surface of the eye

The patient must be encouraged to keep both eyes open. If this is difficult on account of pain or photophobia a drop of short-acting local anaesthetic is invaluable — amethocaine 1% or oxybuprocaine (Benoxinate) 0.4%.

It is usually possible to differentiate redness most marked on the lining of the lids and around the periphery of the eye — conjunctivitis — from that which is duskier in colour and seen mostly around the margin of the cornea — ciliary congestion — implying disease of the cornea, iris, or deeper parts of the eye.

In the examination of the outer eye, the bright shiny surface of the cornea will be noted. Any disturbance of the surface will be demarcated by the use of stain — see above.

Pupils

The pupils should be round, central and of equal size: they should react equally to light and accommodation. Examination requires four simple steps:

1. *Inspection.* Look for any irregularity of size, shape or position of either pupil.

2. *Light reaction.* With the fellow eye covered, shine the brightest light available — it may be a pen torch, ophthalmoscope or a desk light — directly into each eye in turn. A brisk, sustained contraction should be seen, the pupil dilating when the light is removed. The pupil of the eye not exposed to light should constrict to the same extent — this is the consensual reaction.

3. *The swinging light test.* Illuminate first one eye and then the other. Each should show an equal and similarly sustained pupil reaction. Dilation of either pupil when illuminated indicates impaired conduction along the optic nerve on that side — a relative afferent pupillary defect. This is a simple and sensitive test of optic nerve function.

4. *Near response.* The patient is instructed to look in the distance and then at an object held near his face; both pupils should constrict, dilating again when distance fixation is resumed.

Abnormalities are discussed on page 129.

Colour vision

Colour vision testing is sometimes important to the general practitioner. Two circumstances in which assessment can be of value require different equipment:

1. In *optic nerve disorders* (Ch. 14) impaired colour recognition especially of red, is an early finding. Red recognition is easily checked against that of the examiner by the confrontation test described for the visual field (Fig. 5), using a red target. A red topped pin or a small red plastic bottle top are satisfactory. The patient should be asked whether he notices any change of colour of the target, and each eye is compared with that of the examiner.

2. *Congenital colour blindness* occurs in various forms in about 8% of males and 0.4% of females, with sex-linked recessive inheritance. Detection of this defect is useful in routine visual screening, and patients sometimes ask to be tested. Specially designed tests are used in connection with occupational requirements such as for airline and railway staff.

The *Ishihara* test is convenient for the general practitioner. It consists of a book of coloured plates, each bearing a number which the patient has to identify. Plates with wavy lines are provided which can be traced with the finger by illiterate patients. Detailed instructions for the interpretation of incorrect answers are supplied with each book.

Ocular movements

Ocular motility is dealt with in a later chapter, but a complaint of double vision should lead to a test of the ability of the eyes smoothly to follow the movement of an object in various directions, and to find the direction in which double vision is present (see Squint).

The inner eye

Only practice can bring competence with the ophthalmoscope and the ability to recognise abnormalities.

The closer to the eye the instrument is held, the wider the field of view. The use of a plus lens in the ophthalmoscope, and examination at $\frac{1}{3}$ metre, make for easier detection of lens opacities (Fig. 7).

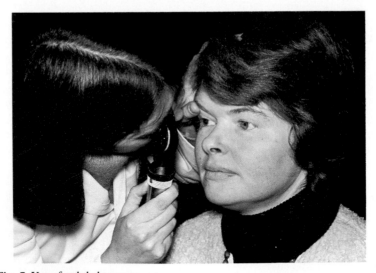

Fig. 7 Use of ophthalmoscope

Of essential importance is the need to examine both eyes, for asymmetry between the eyes is unusual and should make the alarm bells ring. Particularly with regard to the optic disc, differences between the two sides, whether of shape, size, colour, or of the vascular pattern, may be of crucial importance.

It is helpful to have a routine when examining the fundi. One way is to look slightly to the nasal side, focus on a vessel and follow it until the optic disc is seen. The disc is then examined and each of the four main vascular arcades followed peripherally in turn. Finally the macula should be examined; this may require a smaller aperture in the ophthalmoscope if the pupil has not been dilated.

2

Initial assessment

History taking and examination at the first consultation usually point to the nature of the problem. Common presenting symptoms have been discussed in Chapter 1 and the remainder of this book is arranged on an anatomical basis. The purpose of this chapter is to draw the two together.

It must not be forgotten that serious disease of the eye or visual pathway may be present and yet the patient may be unaware of any symptoms.

The situations considered below are:
1. The red eye.
2. Pain attributed to the eye.
3. Sudden visual loss.
4. Gradual visual loss.
5. Distorted vision.
6. Haloes.
7. Flashing lights.
8. Spots before the eye.

1. *The red eye.* Most cases of 'red' eye can be diagnosed and treated at the first visit. Cases of doubt should be referred for initial diagnosis and treatment by an ophthalmologist urgently, if vision is affected (Table 1).

2. *Pain attributed to the eye.* Pain may be due to an ocular disorder or be referred from elsewhere in the head and neck. If it is thought that pain arises in the eye, the general practitioner should refer the patient for urgent examination by an ophthalmologist (Table 2).

3. *Sudden loss of vision.* Visual loss may be total, or partial, affecting only a sector of the visual field: it may be transient, or may persist. Unequivocally diagnosed migraine is the only category in which urgent referral to an ophthalmologist is not mandatory. Patients over 60 who have sudden visual loss must have an immediate ESR or plasma viscosity check to detect asymptomatic giant cell arteritis. Missing this diagnosis may result in visual loss in the second eye and total blindness which could have been prevented.

The principal causes of sudden loss of vision are given in Table 3.

10

Table 1 The red eye

Condition	Symptoms	Signs	Management
Sub-conjunctival haemorrhage (p. 28)	No pain. Normal vision.	Haemorrhage visible. Cornea clear.	No treatment required.
Conjunctivitis (p. 29)	Watery or purulent discharge. Slight or no pain. Normal vision.	Conjunctiva inflamed.	Antibiotic drops if bacterial infection suspected.
Keratitis (p. 48)	Pain and photophobia. Vision impaired if ulcer or opacity near visual axis.	Loss of corneal clarity. Epithelial defect stains with fluorescein.	Antibiotic drops if bacterial infection clearly established — otherwise refer.
Iritis (p. 58)	Pain. Photophobia. Vision may be impaired or increase in floaters.	Small or distorted pupil. Ciliary congestion. Engorged vessels radiating from limbus. Tarsal conjunctiva normal.	Refer for confirmation of initial diagnosis. Treat recurrences with steroid drops and refer for follow-up.
Acute glaucoma (p. 113)	Pain. ± Vomiting. Severe visual impairment. May be bilateral.	Pupil fixed and semidilated. Corneal oedema preventing clear view of iris detail. Shallow anterior chamber. Raised intra-ocular pressure.	Refer urgently.
Episcleritis (p. 35)	Slight or no pain. No discharge. Normal vision.	Localised or diffuse redness of bulbar conjunctiva and underlying episcleral tissues, which may be elevated	Steroid drops, provided cornea is clear. Usually settles without treatment.
Scleritis (p. 35)	Deep-seated pain	Localised or diffuse redness and swelling of sclera. Frequently associated with systemic connective tissue disorder.	Refer.

Each of these conditions is considered in more detail and illustrated in the following chapters.

Table 2 Pain attributed to the eye

	Condition	Features

Major painful eye disorders	Cornea
	  Keratitis (p. 48)
	  Abrasion (p. 46)
	  Foreign body (p. 47)
		Ciliary congestion; fluorescein staining

	Iritis (p. 58)	Ciliary congestion; small, irregular pupil; vision may be impaired
	Scleritis (p. 35)	Usually associated systemic disorder
	Acute glaucoma (p. 113)	Corneal oedema; fixed, semi-dilated pupil; shallow anterior chamber; hard eye; may be vomiting

Eye disorders causing discomfort	Lids
	  Entropion (p. 20)
	  Trichiasis (p. 19)
		Malpositioned or loose lashes

	Conjunctiva Conjunctivitis (p. 29)	Palpebral and bulbar conjunctiva inflamed; discharge
	Dry eye (p. 25)	Rose bengal punctate staining; Schirmer's test
	Episcleritis (p. 35)	Nodular or diffuse
	Optic neuritis (p. 124)	Vision impaired; colour recognition defective; afferent pupillary defect; discomfort on palpating globe and lateral gaze; may be disc swelling

Pain referred to the eye	Trigeminal nerve
	  Herpes zoster
	  ophthalmicus
	  (p. 51)
		Rash

	Trigeminal neuralgia	Lancinating pain; trigger zone
	Sinusitis	Tender on pressure over sinus; X-ray
	Scalp (p. 123) Giant cell arteritis	Tenderness; raised ESR/plasma viscosity; may lead to sudden visual loss (ischaemic optic neuropathy)
	Neck Tension headache	Continuous, symmetrical pain; not associated with visual or gastrointestinal symptoms
	Intracranial Migraine	Aura; distribution; duration; gastrointestinal symptoms
	Migrainous neuralgia	'Cluster' incidence; unilateral; associated lacrimal and nasal discharge
	Raised intra-cranial pressure (p. 126)	Papilloedema; nausea/vomiting; headache worse in morning and on coughing/straining
	Intra-cranial aneurysm	Associated cranial nerve lesion
	Refractive error (p. 98)	Symptoms suggest eyestrain
	Ocular muscle imbalance (p. 103)	Refer for refraction in first instance

Table 3 Sudden loss of vision

Site	Cause	Features
Vitreous	Massive vitreous haemorrhage (p. 76)	Loss of red reflex on fundus examination
Retina	Retinal arterial occlusion (p. 73)	Branch — partial loss of vision. Central — total loss of vision and of direct pupillary reaction.
	Central retinal vein occlusion (p. 74)	Extensive haemorrhage in fundus
	Amaurosis fugax (p. 74)	'Curtain' over vision, usually recovering in minutes. Embolus may be visible in retinal arteriole.
	Retinal detachment involving macula (p. 84)	History of flashing lights and peripheral loss extending to central field
Optic nerve	Ischaemic optic neuropathy (p. 123)	a. Arteriosclerotic — usually partial visual loss and disc swelling b. Giant cell arteritis — disc swelling. ESR/viscosity raised.
	Toxic amblyopia (p. 78)	Quinine or methyl alcohol poisoning
Visual pathway	Stroke (p. 128)	Homonymous hemianopia (the patient may think it unilateral). Total visual loss if previous hemianopia unrecognised or cortical blindness. Normal pupil reactions.
	Migraine	Characteristic aura and recovery. Scintillating scotoma; flashing lights. Gastrointestinal symptoms. Recovery almost invariable.
Acute glaucoma (p. 113)		Pain ± vomiting. Red eye. Corneal oedema. Semi-dilated pupil. Eye stony hard.

NB Apparently sudden visual loss may be due to the discovery of a pre-existing defect or to hysteria. Referral is always justified.

4. *Gradual loss of vision.* Many disorders of the eye or visual pathway result in gradual loss of vision. The commonest are given in Table 4.

Table 4 Gradual loss of vision

	Cause	Features
Lens	Cataract (p. 66)	Increased myopia or blurring
Retina	Macular degeneration (p. 77)	Straight lines appear distorted. Peripheral field unaffected
	Retinal vein occlusion (p. 74)	Typical retinal haemorrhages
	Retinal detachment (p. 84)	Flashing lights, and floaters. Increasing field loss and central visual loss later
Optic nerve	Chronic glaucoma (p. 114)	Usually so gradual as to pass unnoticed. Optic disc cupping, raised intra-ocular pressure and field loss
	Optic neuritis (p. 124)	Age group 20–45. Central visual defect — peripheral field intact. Eye tender on palpation and looking sideways. Impaired direct pupillary light reaction (p. 7) Spontaneous recovery usual in 2–4 weeks
	Toxic optic neuropathy (p. 125).	Heavy smoking and/or alcohol intake. Peripheral field intact
Visual pathway	Compressive lesions of visual pathway	Must be excluded if other causes not found. Temporal field defect usual. Lateral X-ray of pituitary fossa is the minimum investigation

5. *Distorted central vision* may be due to:

a. Retinal detachment beginning to involve macula (p. 84).

b. Macular degeneration of any type (p. 77).

c. Macular haemorrhage.

Pupillary light reaction is normal. Dilation of the pupil is essential for satisfactory examination.

6. *Haloes round lights* may be due to:

a. Raised intra-ocular pressure in angle-closure glaucoma (p. 113).

b. Corneal disease.

c. Lens opacities.
Always refer for investigation to exclude angle-closure glaucoma.

7. *Flashing lights* before one or both eyes — the patient may not
be sure — may be due to:
a. Scintillating scotoma of migraine.
b. Retinal tear (p. 85)
c. Retinal detachment (p. 85)
d. Vitreous detachment.
Unless the history of migraine is certain, refer for detailed retinal
examination by an ophthalmologist.

8. *Spots before the eyes* may be due to:
a. Vitreous haemorrhage — any cause (p. 76)
b. Uveitis with vitreous opacities (p. 60)
c. Retinal tear with operculum lying in the vitreous (p. 85).
d. Posterior vitreous detachment occurring suddenly, with or without associated retinal tear or detachment (p. 84).
e. 'Innocent' degenerative changes in the vitreous (p. 70).
This list contains enough vision-threatening conditions to justify
referral if the general practitioner is not entirely satisfied the
condition is due to innocent vitreous floaters and there are no factors
predisposing to retinal detachment.

Flashing light *and* spots before the eyes are a particularly dangerous combination — referral essential.

REFERRALS

Except in cases of emergency, when contact is likely to be made
by telephone, the majority of patients referred will have been examined initially by an optician.

The sight-testing optician, when suggesting that the general practitioner be consulted, will send a letter or completed pro-forma to
the doctor. This report contains details of the optician's reasons for
doubt and it or a photocopy should be sent complete to the ophthalmologist with the referral letter.

The optician's report will record the visual acuity, the spectacle
correction and any other findings. If this information is available
to the ophthalmologist, unnecessary repetition of some tests will be
avoided and the point of the optician's referral will not be missed.

Also of importance are details of the patient's general state of health, with information about relevant past illnesses and family history. These are especially helpful with elderly patients who may not be good historians. A recent blood pressure reading and the result of a urine test for glucose will also be much appreciated.

3

The eyelids

ANATOMY

The skin of the eyelids is thin and there is no subcutaneous fat. This accounts for the ready swelling that accompanies any inflammatory or traumatic condition.

In the normal position, the margin of the upper lid crosses the upper third of the cornea, while the lower lid margin lies at the lower limbus (junction of cornea and sclera). Exposure of sclera below the cornea is one of the first signs of proptosis.

The tarsal or Meibomian glands lie in the substance of the lid and discharge at the lid margin.

At the anterior part of their free margins, the lids have two or three rows of lashes, but the inner end of each lid is free of lashes and carries the lacrimal punctum, the upper end of the lacrimal drainage apparatus. The punctum is directed backwards toward the globe and cannot be seen unless the lid is everted.

The orbicularis oculi, supplied by the facial nerve, forms a circle round the orbit and is responsible for blinking and for the forcible protective closure seen in injury or inflammation. The levator of the upper lid is supplied by a branch of the third cranial nerve.

WOUNDS OF THE LIDS

These injuries demand special attention, not only because of the risks associated with improper handling, but also because they may accompany an injury to the eyeball. Lid wounds are best treated in a specialist unit, as the distortion resulting from incorrect alignment may lead to unsightly notching of the lid margin, misdirection of the lashes or interference with the lacrimal drainage apparatus.

Destructive injuries of the lids present a risk of exposure of the cornea. On no account must the cornea be allowed to become dry.

Pending repair, the cornea should be protected, either by the use of plenty of ointment and a pad, or by two or three temporary stitches to hold the torn lids over the globe.

INFLAMMATION OF THE LIDS

Blepharitis (inflammation of the lid margins) (Plate 1)

There is a complaint of chronically irritable eyes; the lid margins are reddened and conjunctivitis is present. Fine crusts are seen at the roots of the lashes and seborrhoea capitis seems to be a common association. Treatment is tedious and often unrewarding. Crusts must be removed with a cotton 'bud' soaked in a bland solution each morning during active phases. Antibiotic ointment at bedtime may be a help, with a short course of combined antibiotic–steroid for exacerbations if necessary.

Hordeolum (stye)

An abscess in one of the glands related to a lash follicle. Pointing, therefore, occurs in the line of the lashes, distinguishing this condition from the chalazion.

Treat by hot bathing and antibiotic ointment.

SWELLINGS OF THE LID

Benign

Chalazion (meibomian cyst)

A chronic swelling in the substance of the lid, painless unless abscess formation occurs. Characteristically centred some distance from the lid margin and thus distinguished from a stye (Plate 2).

Chalazia are often multiple and repeated, and are common in association with rosacea.

Treatment consists of curettage of the cyst through a small vertical incision on the conjunctival surface of the lid. This is an outpatient procedure.

Other cysts

Sebaceous cysts and molluscum contagiosum need surgical evacuation.

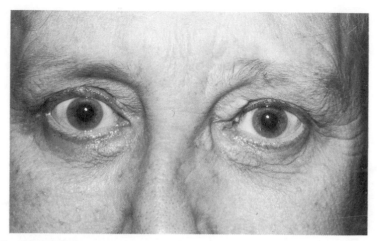

Fig. 8 Xanthelasma

Xanthelasma (Fig. 8)

Common in the elderly and in diabetics, these flat creamy plaques may be removed on cosmetic grounds. They may signify hyperlipidaemia.

Malignant

Basal-cell carcinoma (rodent ulcer) (Plate 3)

Characteristic rolled edges; typically seen in Europeans who have been exposed over many years to bright sunlight. The commonest malignancy in the eyelid: slow-growing and only locally invasive. If untreated, it leads to considerable loss of tissue. Treatment is by surgical excision with 2 mm of surrounding tissue, radiotherapy or cryotherapy, depending on the size and situation of the lesion.

Squamous carcinoma (epithelioma)

Requires wide excision after diagnostic biopsy.

MALPOSITIONS OF THE LID

Trichiasis

Although the normal position of the lid is not disturbed, trichiasis implies maldirection of the eyelashes. This may result from wounds or from inflammation, and may affect a single lash follicle or many. The abnormal lashes rub against the globe, with resultant irritation, watering and potential damage to the cornea.

Treatment is difficult. A single lash can usually be pulled out but trichiasis involving many lashes is often an intractable problem. Electrolysis may be helpful.

Entropion (Fig. 9)

A backward rolling of the lid edge, with the lashes actually disappearing from view, occurs mostly in the elderly and is a result of spasm of the inner fibres of the orbicularis oculi (senile spastic entropion).

The condition may occur spontaneously or follow some irritative condition of the eye. The eye may appear normal on examination though the entropion can often be induced by asking the patient to close the eye forcibly. Temporary relief can be obtained by the use of a strip of plaster between the lid and the cheek, but recurrent or persistent entropion needs surgical repair.

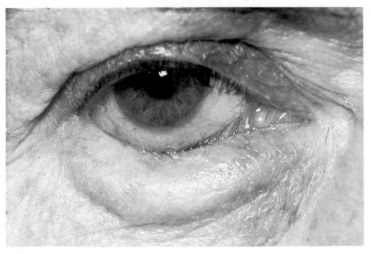

Fig. 9 Entropion

Ectropion (Fig. 10)

The edge of the lid may fall away from the eye as a result of contracture from wounds or inflammation, but it is most common as a result of loss of tone in the facial muscles.

The inner end of the lid being first involved, the principal complaint will be of watering, but later there will be conjunctivitis and increased discharge.

Treatment is surgical, but the patient should be taught not to make the condition worse by wiping his eyes downwards. He should wipe his eye upwards and medially towards the nose.

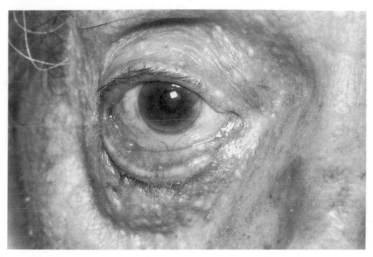

Fig. 10 Ectropion

Ptosis (Fig. 11)

Drooping of the upper lid is a feature of palsy of the third cranial nerve and thus may result from a multitude of neurological conditions. It is a diagnostic sign of myasthenia gravis, in which it can be induced or made worse by asking the patient to gaze steadily at a finger held in front of his face and above the horizontal plane.

Of greater importance from the ophthalmic point of view is congenital ptosis, unilateral or bilateral, complete or partial, and often associated with limited elevation of the affected eye, from weakness of the superior rectus muscle. It is impossible to mistake the child suffering from bilateral congenital ptosis, with the characteristic 'head-back' attitude in his attempt to see through the reduced palpebral aperture.

Treatment is surgical, and the timing of the operation depends on the child's age and whether or not there is a risk of the eye becoming amblyopic ('lazy') from disuse.

Congenital ptosis is often associated with epicanthus, a prominent

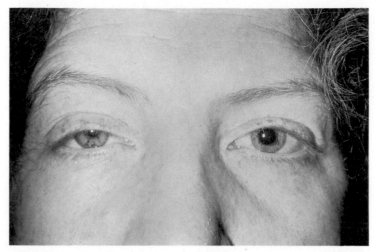

Fig. 11 Ptosis in Horner's syndrome (see also p. 129)

fold of skin overlying the inner corner of the eye. Improvement in this usually takes place as the child grows.

Senile ptosis is not uncommon: surgery may be indicated.

DRUG SENSITIVITY REACTIONS

Allergic conjunctivitis with dermatitis involving the skin around the eyelids sometimes occurs when substances to which the patient is allergic are applied locally. Plate 4 illustrates such a reaction to atropine; excess drops can be seen to have run down the patient's cheek. Other drugs, notably neomycin and sulphacetamide, and some cosmetics may cause a similar reaction. Treatment consists of withdrawing the offending substance. The intense irritation may be relieved by 1% hydrocortisone lotion.

FACIAL PALSY

Idiopathic facial palsy (Bell's palsy) may lead to exposure keratitis. In the early stage this is best prevented by applying ointment — usually containing an antibiotic such as chloramphenicol — liberally to the eye at night. If the eye becomes inflamed or corneal staining with fluorescein can be demonstrated, the patient should be referred. Joining the lids by lateral tarsorrhaphy protects the cornea.

4

Lacrimal system

ANATOMY AND PHYSIOLOGY

The lacrimal gland lies in the upper outer corner of the orbit and its secretion drains into the upper conjunctival fornix. From here the tears are carried by the movements of the lids toward the inner corner of the eye. On each lid, close to the inner end, is a minute lacrimal punctum. It cannot be seen until the lid is everted, for it normally is directed backwards towards the globe.

From the puncta two canaliculi carry the tears medially to the lacrimal sac, out of which the naso-lacrimal duct drains into the inferior meatus of the nose.

In addition to the lacrimal gland, the conjunctiva has mucous and accessory lacrimal glands, which keep the conjunctiva and cornea moist. Secretion of the lacrimal gland itself only occurs under conditions of irritation or emotion.

THE WATERY EYE

Abnormal watering of the eye is caused either by overproduction of tears or interference with outflow.

Epiphora from overproduction of tears

1. Irritation of conjunctiva or cornea. May result from a conjunctival or corneal foreign body, or conjunctivitis.
2. Reflex epiphora from irritation of the fifth cranial nerve. Also, in some people, from exposure to bright light.
3. Emotion.

Epiphora from failure of outflow

Interference with the punctum

There may be congenital absence of the punctum: it may be everted

and thus fail to pick up the tears from the conjunctival sac, or stenosis may follow inflammation or wounds of the lid.

Occasionally, a loose lash gets washed into the punctum, giving
rise to a characteristic patch of redness where it rubs against the
conjunctiva. Removal of the lash produces a gratifyingly rapid cure.

Obstruction in the canaliculus

Canalicular blockage is a common cause of epiphora: it sometimes
follows trauma. The results of surgical treatment are disappointing.

Obstruction in the naso-lacrimal duct

1. In infancy. This is the commonest cause of unilateral conjunctivitis in a baby.

The naso-lacrimal drainage apparatus develops from a solid cord
of ectodermal cells folded into the face along the groove between
the fronto-nasal and maxillary processes. Subsequent canalisation
leads to the formation of the lacrimal sac and naso-lacrimal duct.
In some cases canalisation is incomplete, or an accumulation of cast-
off epithelial cells and debris blocks the duct.

There is no abnormality during the first few weeks of life, and
then the eye becomes watery and tends to be sticky. Finger pressure
over the lacrimal sac may produce a reflux of mucoid material from
the punctum.

Conservative treatment is worthwhile for a few weeks. The
child's mother is instructed to keep the sac empty by finger pressure
several times a day, antibiotic drops being used at the same time.
Many cases resolve spontaneously, but failure to do so is an indication for probing of the duct. This is done as an out-patient procedure under general anaesthetic.

2. In the adult. Chronic obstruction of the naso-lacrimal duct
often is due to dacryocystitis, more common in women than in men,
and mostly after the menopause.

Chronic dacryocystitis leads to constant watering of the eye and
may be associated with the development of a mucocele from
which muco-pus can be expressed by finger pressure over the sac.

Not only is the obstructed duct liable to acute inflammation, it
is also a reservoir from which infected material is constantly entering the conjunctival sac. This means that any injury to the eye is
liable to become infected, and any operation is similarly at risk.

In most cases the treatment is the creation of a new channel to the nose. Dacryocystorhinostomy (DCR) consists of making an anastomosis between the lacrimal and nasal mucous membranes. This allows the tears to enter the nose, bypassing the obstructed nasolacrimal duct.

Drops containing zinc sulphate 0.25% and a decongestant (Zincfrin) are sometimes helpful in giving symptomatic relief, used on a 'p.r.n.' basis. But they have no effect on the underlying lacrimal obstruction and must be used with caution in eyes in which the anterior chamber is shallow, on account of the risk of angle closure glaucoma.

THE DRY EYE

Inadequate tear production is an important cause of ocular discomfort and contributes to many cases of failure to tolerate contact lenses. It is common in healthy individuals in its milder forms. Tear secretion naturally decreases with advancing age. The patient complains of vague irritation and attacks of redness of the eyes. The symptoms are variable, and tend to be worst in centrally heated buildings without adequate humidification, and travelling in cars with the heater blowing hot air.

Patients with collagen disorders, particularly rheumatoid arthritis, are prone to a more severe form of kerato-conjunctivitis sicca, characterised by diminished tear and salivary secretion, with dryness of the cornea and formation of filaments on its surface (Sjogren's syndrome).

The tear production can be assessed by Schirmer's test (Fig. 12). A strip of filter paper 5 mm wide is placed over the margin of the lower lid, and removed after 5 minutes. The length of the strip wetted by the tears is measured: 15 mm or more indicates normal tear production.

Rose bengal staining (obtainable in Minims) of the cornea and conjunctiva is another method of assessing the adequacy of tear secretion. Dry eyes show multiple punctate epithelial defects when examined under magnification with a loupe (p. 1).

Although defective tear production cannot be cured, symptomatic relief can be achieved by the use of artificial tear supplements. Methyl cellulose 0.5 or 1% drops have stood the test of time, but there are numerous proprietary tear supplements: they can be purchased by patients without prescription. Frequency of use varies with the degree of symptoms.

Patients whose dry eyes cause distress in spite of the use of ar-

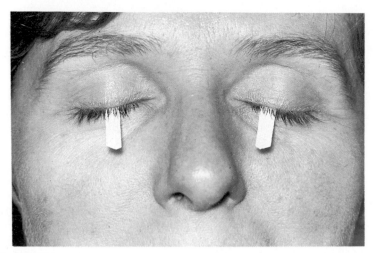

Fig. 12 Schirmers test

tificial tears may be helped by surgical occlusion of the lacrimal puncta to conserve tears. Soft, 'bandage' contact lenses, lubricated by a tear supplement, may also give relief.

Dry eye problems which do not respond to simple measures should be referred for specialist assessment.

5

Conjunctiva and sclera

ANATOMY

The conjunctiva is a thin mucous membrane covering the anterior portion of the eyeball (bulbar conjunctiva) and lining the lids (palpebral conjunctiva).

It contains numerous glands which moisten the surface — goblet cells and accessory lacrimal glands. Lubrication is also provided by the lacrimal gland. Tears contain lysozyme which, by its bacteriostatic action, inhibits the multiplication of organisms in the warm, moist conjunctival sac.

Deep to the conjunctiva is the tough sclera, composed of collagen, blending with the cornea at the limbus.

CONJUNCTIVA

Injuries to the conjunctiva

Lacerations

Conjunctival lacerations require to be treated with greater respect than their apparent simplicity suggests, for there may be a concealed penetration of the eyeball. An attempt must be made to assess the visual acuity of the injured eye and to examine the eye with an ophthalmoscope. Neither is likely to be easy in the case of a child, or in the presence of a painful corneal abrasion, but should not be omitted on this account. The conjunctiva heals rapidly if the wound edges are in apposition but gaping wounds should be repaired to avoid the formation of granulation tissue.

If there is doubt about the integrity of the eye, refer immediately.

Conjunctival foreign bodies

Foreign bodies blown into the eye, or loose lashes, commonly lodge in the lower fornix and are easily removed while the patient looks

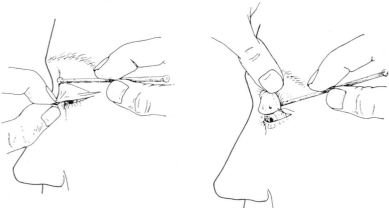

Fig. 13 Eversion of upper lid

upwards. If the particle lies beneath the upper lid, not only does it scratch the cornea with each blink, but it cannot be removed without everting the lid to expose its under surface.

The steps are as follows (Fig. 13):

1. The patient looks downwards with both eyes open.
2. The operator grasps the lashes between finger and thumb of one hand while, with the other, he presses with the tip of a pencil, glass rod or matchstick on the skin of the lid just above the tarsal plate.
3. The foreign body is removed.
4. It is wise to stain the cornea with fluorescein (p. 2). If an abrasion is found, antibiotic ointment should be instilled and a firm pad applied for the remainder of the day.

The upper and lower fornices of the conjunctival sac are surprisingly capacious, and quite large foreign bodies such as air gun pellets may be concealed in them.

Subconjunctival haemorrhage (Plate 5)

A localised haemorrhage may follow contusion to the eye and often is part of an orbital haematoma. The haemorrhage is absorbed in a week or two, but, if severe, it should raise suspicion of more serious injury such as fracture of the orbital walls, or penetrating injury of the globe. It should also be remembered that orbital haemorrhage may result from remote injury to the skull and follow subarachnoid haemorrhage.

Spontaneous subconjunctival haemorrhages, which are often recurrent, are common in the elderly and may be a manifestation of hypertension or generalised arteriosclerosis. The patient needs reassurance only.

Chemical injuries of the conjunctiva

Energetic first aid may have a great influence on the ultimate result of injury to the eye by corrosive chemicals.

Workers in chemical industries or laboratories may receive splashes of liquid acids or alkalis in the eyes. Although reflex tear production dilutes the irritant, immediate irrigation of the eyes with abundant water may be a sight-saving measure. The injured person's head should be held under a tap, and companions should help to hold the eyes open while water runs over them. The subsequent management depends on the severity of the burning and the nature of the chemical concerned. Alkalis are in general more dangerous than acids. Liquid ammonia and caustic soda cause permanent corneal and conjunctival damage and maybe blindness. Any severe case should be referred after immediate first aid.

Lime requires special mention. Lime particles may be splashed in the face, especially in building workers, through powder flying up in careless mixing of cement. There is immediate blepharospasm and lacrimation, making examination difficult.

Treatment is as follows:
1. Anaesthetise with 1% amethocaine.
2. Remove all solid particles of lime from the conjunctiva, using forceps or cotton wool swabs.
3. Irrigate the eye thoroughly with water.
4. Stain the cornea with fluorescein.
5. If the cornea is clear and there is no evidence of conjunctival necrosis in the fornices, instil antibiotic ointment.
6 If necrosis is present or the cornea hazy, refer.

Conjunctivitis

Inflammation of the conjunctiva is the commonest ophthalmic problem requiring treatment by the general practitioner. It may be of any degree of severity.

Symptoms are discomfort, discharge and difficulty opening the eye on waking.

Table 5 Causes of conjunctivitis

Cause	Clinical features
Bacterial infections (see Table 6)	Mucopurulent discharge, crusting on lashes
Viral infection	Non-purulent. ± lower fornix follicles ±corneal lesions No response to antibiotics
Allergy Atopic conjunctivitis	Marked in pollen season History of allergy Itching the main symptom
Vernal conjunctivitis	Papillae — upper tarsal conjunctiva ± corneal lesions
Chemical and drug reactions	History of exposure ± lower fornix follicles
Mechanical causes	Eyelid abnormalities Trichiasis Exposure
Dry eye	Rose bengal staining Reduced Schirmer test result ± associated systemic disorder

Table 6 Bacteria commonly causing conjunctivitis

Haemophilus influenzae
Streptococcus pneumoniae
Moraxella lacunata
Staphylococcus aureus

Signs are redness and discharge adherent to the lashes. Hypertrophy of *lymphoid follicles* should be noted, particularly in the lower fornix where they appear as shiny round swellings and of *papillae* which, under magnification, can be seen to have vessels at their centre. The upper lid should be everted to look for enlarged papillae on its conjunctival surface. Pre-auricular lymph node enlargement should be noted. Visual acuity is not affected unless there is also corneal involvement, but the cornea should be stained with fluorescein and examined with magnification and a good light (see p. 2) to ensure that the epithelium is intact.

Some cases of chronic conjunctivitis defy definitive diagnosis and effective therapy. Such patients may be referred for assessment by an ophthalmologist.

Bacterial conjunctivitis (Plate 6)

Purulent discharge and difficulty opening the eyes on waking are the cardinal features, with relatively mild, gritty discomfort. It is helpful, but not essential, to take a bacterial culture before starting treatment. The result may be available by the time the patient returns if the initial treatment does not prove satisfactory.

Antibiotic drops — usually chloramphenicol or neomycin — should be given for at least 5 days: ointment at night may be given in addition.

Chlamydial conjunctivitis (Plate 7)

Bacteria of the genus Chlamydia live only within cells, forming intracellular inclusion bodies. *Chlamydia trachomatis* affects the human eye and genital tract. Following an acute initial infection a chronic, often sub-clinical phase usually follows.

Three distinct clinical syndromes are produced by infection of the conjunctiva by *C. trachomatis*:

1. *Neonatal inclusion conjunctivitis* (see p. 32).

2. *Endemic trachoma* — a chronic infection seen amongst underprivileged people living in warm dry climates with poor standards of hygiene. It is the world's major blinding condition. Sporadic cases seen in developed countries are usually inactive, but where there is doubt, patients should be referred for assessment by an ophthalmologist.

3. *C. trachomatis conjunctivitis* (adult inclusion conjunctivitis) is caused by strains of this organism which infect the genital tract and are transmitted to the eye following sexual contact. Sexually active adults are affected and the resulting conjunctivitis is florid, predominantly in the lower fornix, with follicle formation and punctate staining of the cornea.

The *diagnosis* is usually made clinically after the condition has failed to respond to conventional treatment for bacterial conjunctivitis. A special transport medium is needed for the successful culture of the organism. Microscopic examination of conjunctival scrapings for inclusion bodies may help confirm the diagnosis.

Treatment. A 3-week course of tetracycline ointment and oral erythromycin 250 mg four times a day is usually sufficient to eliminate both the conjunctival and genital infection. Inquiry should be made about sexual contacts and these should be referred for treatment by the general practitioner or venereologist.

Conjunctivitis in the newborn (Ophthalmia neonatorum)

This is a notifiable disease and the definition includes any case of purulent discharge from the eyes of a child occurring within 21 days of birth.

Infection occurs during passage through an infected birth canal and usually appears within 2 or 3 days as gross oedema of the lids, between which pus escapes when an attempt is made to open the eye. The conjunctiva is seen to be congested and swollen (chemosis). The organisms commonly found on culture are listed in Table 7.

Table 7 Pathogens found in neonatal conjunctivitis

Pathogen	Recommended first antibiotic
N. gonorrhoeae Staph. aureus Strep. pneumoniae Haemophilus spp.	Oc. chloramphenicol until sensitivities are known
Chlamydia trachomatis	Oc. tetracycline for baby. Tabs erythromycin for mother

A culture should be taken from any newborn infant with conjunctivitis and the eyes should be examined to determine the state of the cornea. Initial treatment with chloramphenicol ointment six times daily normally clears the infection. If there is any question of corneal damage or the infection persists, viral cultures should also be taken. Discharge must be removed as it forms. Treatment is best carried out in hospital.

Viral conjunctivitis

Adenovirus. Typically occurring in epidemics, eye infection by adenovirus is a potentially serious, bilateral condition. There is nonpurulent, watery discharge. The conjunctivitis is associated with fine, punctate corneal ulcers and sub-epithelial opacities and frequently, pre-auricular lymph node enlargement. The diagnosis can be confirmed by culture using a virus transport medium. The symptoms may persist for months or years with episodes of recurrence.

Strict hygienic precautions must be observed to minimise the risk of transfer of infection, especially at school and within the family.

Treatment is of little value, though symptomatic relief may be obtained from agents containing vasoconstrictors. Patients in whom corneal complications are suspected should be referred for specialist care.

Herpes simplex. Primary herpes simplex infection may cause a short-lived conjunctivitis. Herpes simplex keratitis is discussed on page 50.

Herpes zoster. The affected eye may show marked conjunctival involvement. Management is discussed on page 51.

Other virus infections. Transient non-purulent conjunctivitis is a feature of many systemic viral infections. No specific treatment is required, the watering and redness settling with the resolution of the illness.

Allergic conjunctivitis

Allergic conjunctivitis occurs in several distinct forms:

1. *Acute conjunctival chemosis* (oedema). This bilateral condition may develop with dramatic suddenness and disappear equally quickly. Treatment, apart from identifying and if possible avoiding the cause, is with topical or oral antihistamines. 'Otrivine Antistine' drops instilled every hour or two until the swelling subsides usually prove satisfactory.

2. *Chronic allergic conjunctivitis.* Usually a mild, bilateral inflammation with marked itching and no discharge: follicles may be present. It occurs most during the hay fever season. Treatment with antihistamines such as 'Otrivine Antistine' or with sodium cromoglycate (Opticrom) usually gives relief. More severe cases may be treated with short courses of topical steroid — combined with antibiotic if bacterial infection is thought to coexist — provided the integrity of the corneal epithelium has been established by staining with fluorescein and careful examination.

Patients with persistent allergic conjunctivitis may be helped by investigation of underlying allergies and appropriate desensitisation.

3. *Vernal conjunctivitis* ('Spring catarrh'). Typically seen in atopic individuals in childhood and early adult life, the most serious of these IgE mediated conditions is readily diagnosed by the finding of cobblestone-like giant papillae in the upper tarsal conjunctiva of both eyes on everting the upper lids (Plate 8).

Numerous eosinophils are found on microscopic examination of the conjunctival scrapings. Corneal ulceration and plaque-formation are common complications. Once diagnosed, the condition should be managed under specialist care, but the general practitioner may have to handle periodic exacerbations. Topical steroids such as prednisolone 0.5% drops and sodium cromoglycate (Opticrom) are of about equal effectiveness. The condition usually resolves in early adult life, but permanent corneal scarring may remain.

4. *Drug-induced dermato-conjunctivitis* (see p. 22 and Plate 4).

Chronic non-specific conjunctivitis. Conjunctivitis which persists despite treatment is common, though seldom disabling. Abnormalities of the eyelids — ectropion and entropion — and trichiasis should be excluded and tear secretion measured by Schirmer's test (p. 25). Referral of these patients to an ophthalmologist seldom results in a curative prescription, but useful reassurance may be obtained.

Degenerative conditions of the conjunctiva

Pinguecula (Plate 9)

This is a common condition in adults of all ages. Near the corneoscleral junction medially and laterally, areas of sub-conjunctival degeneration occur, seen as creamy triangular plaques which may be elevated. Occasionally pingueculae become inflamed. Steroid drops remove the redness but the usual precautions of staining the cornea to exclude ulceration and avoidance of prolonged use of the drops must be observed.

Pterygium (Plate 10)

A wing-like area of sub-conjunctival degeneration occurs at the limbus and extends over the cornea. An opaque zone preceding the tip of the advancing pterygium indicates activity. If it is considered unsightly or threatens to cover the pupil the patient should be referred for excision of the pterygium. A few days of considerable discomfort usually follow excision and recurrence is possible. The patient should be warned of this.

Tumours of the conjunctiva

These are rare and include the following:

Benign

Papillomata and *cysts* may be simply excised if causing discomfort or cosmetic blemish.

Naevus

Often close to the limbus, a conjunctival mole may be of any colour from coffee to jet black. It is slightly raised and has a nodular surface. Some become larger or darker at puberty. Unless excision is demanded for cosmetic reasons, no treatment is indicated. Any increase in size or vascularity of the lesion — like melanomata elsewhere — should be regarded with suspicion. Malignant change occurs rarely and is an indication for wide excision.

Malignant

Carcinoma: very rare. *Malignant melanoma*: see above.

EPISCLERA

Episcleritis (Plate 11)

Inflammation of the episcleral tissue deep to the conjunctiva is usually unilateral, with slight discomfort but no discharge. The eye many be diffusely red or the inflammation localised: there may be an inflamed nodule, usually in the inter-palpebral zone. The adjacent conjunctiva is not inflamed.

Although episcleritis may be associated with systemic disorders, it usually occurs for no known reason in healthy individuals. It tends to resolve spontaneously in a few weeks, but this may be hastened by treatment with steroid drops such as prednisolone 0.5% four times daily until the eye is white. It is important to ensure that the cornea does not stain with fluorescein before starting treatment with steroids.

SCLERA

Scleritis (Plate 12)

Inflammation of the sclera is painful and may affect both eyes. The deeper scleral vessels are seen to be engorged. Prolonged scleritis leads to scleral thinning so that the blue of the underlying ciliary body is seen. There may be associated sclerosis of the adjacent cornea leading to opacification or marginal corneal thinning. Perforation of the eye is rare.

Scleritis is usually seen in association with significant systemic disease — most commonly rheumatoid arthritis complicated by vasculitis, which may be visible elsewhere. The overall incidence of scleritis in rheumatoid patients is less than 0.5%

Treatment of scleritis is initially a matter for a specialist. Systemic medication is required as eye drops are usually ineffective, except for associated iritis. Management may be prolonged and co-operation is usually needed between general practitioner, ophthalmologist and specialist physician or rheumatologist.

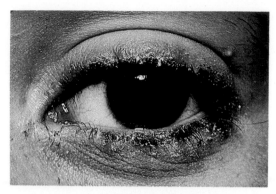

Plate 1 Blepharitis

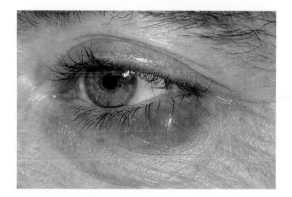

Plate 2 Tarsal cyst (chalazion)

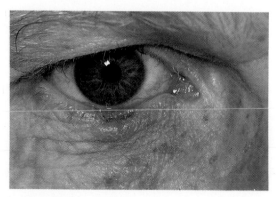

Plate 3 Basal cell carcinoma

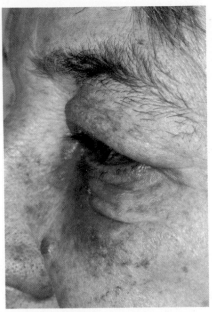

Plate 4 Drug reaction (atropine drops)

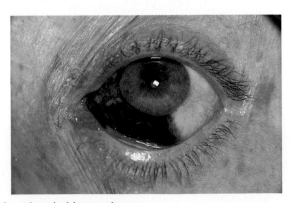

Plate 5 Sub-conjunctival haemorrhage

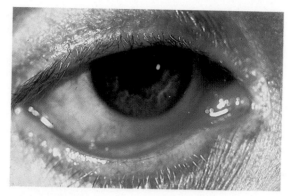

Plate 6 Bacterial conjunctivitis

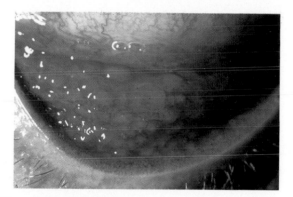

Plate 7 Chlamydial conjunctivitis

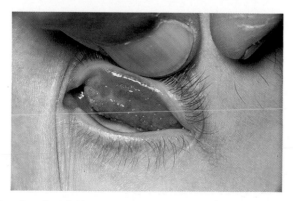

Plate 8 Vernal conjunctivitis

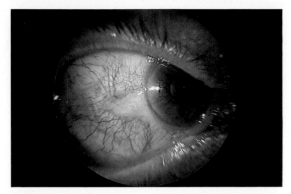

Plate 9 Pinguecula

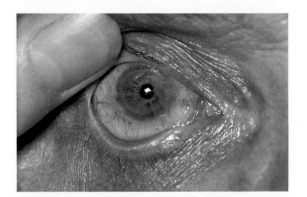

Plate 10 Pterygium

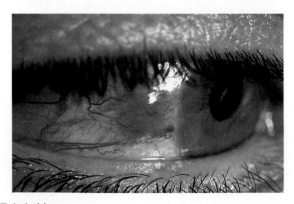

Plate 11 Episcleritis

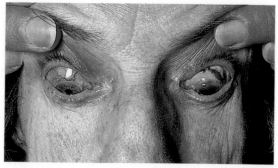

Plate 12 Scleritis (right eye, active stage; left eye, scleral thinning)

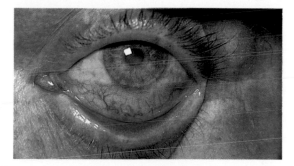

Plate 13 Corneal abrasion stained with fluorescein

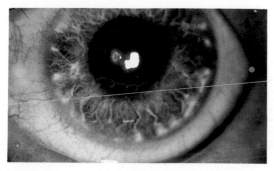

Plate 14 Dendritic ulcer stained with fluorescein

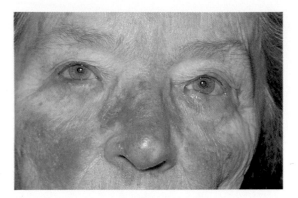

Plate 15 Rosacea

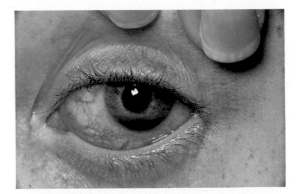

Plate 16 Traumatic hyphaema

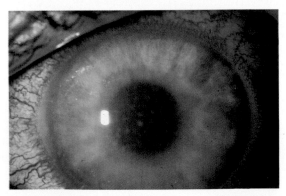

Plate 17 Iritis (note ciliary and iris vessel congestion and keratic precipitates)

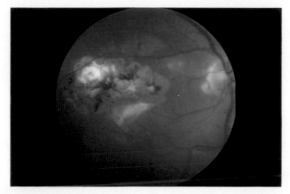

Plate 18 Toxoplasmosis

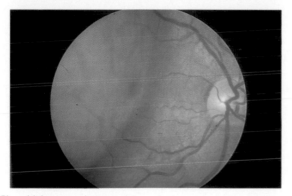

Plate 19 Choroidal tumour (metastatic)

6

The cornea

ANATOMY

The cornea is the transparent anterior portion of the outer coat of the eye. Despite its relative thinness (about 1 mm), the cornea is remarkably tough and the risk of penetrating the eye during removal of a foreign body is negligible. The exposed surface of the cornea is covered with epithelium continuous with that of the conjunctiva. Beneath the epithelium are numerous *free nerve endings* which account for the extreme sensitivity of the cornea to touch and the pain resulting from corneal injury or inflammation.

The stroma of the cornea is bounded superficially by *Bowman's membrane* and on its deep surface by *Descemet's membrane*. The innermost layer, deep to Descemet's membrane, is the *endothelium*. This single layer of cells is important in keeping the cornea optically clear by the transfer of fluid from the stroma into the adjacent anterior chamber against the hydrostatic gradient of the intra-ocular pressure. The endothelium is of great importance to the surgeon carrying out intra-ocular procedures as its cells do not regenerate; they enlarge to cover a greater area as their number diminishes owing to ageing, disease or trauma. Should they fail to maintain corneal clarity, corneal oedema develops and vision is lost.

At the periphery the cornea blends with the sclera at the limbus — a specialised region where most of the drainage of aqueous humour takes place. The inner aspect of this area has a specialised structure, the *trabecular meshwork*, communicating via the *canal of Schlemm* with the episcleral veins on the surface of the globe.

CONGENITAL AND HEREDITARY DISEASE

Keratoconus (conical cornea)

The cornea, having been normal in childhood, gradually loses its normal curvature and becomes increasingly steeply curved, with

44

resultant irregular refraction of the entering light. Visual acuity falls, usually during early adult life, and cannot be adequately improved by spectacles. No medical treatment can arrest this process, but satisfactory vision can often be achieved with hard contact lenses (see p. 99). If corneal scarring or oedema develop, vision may be restored by corneal grafting. Keratoconus is more commonly seen in atopic individuals. It can most easily be demonstrated by observing the lower lid curvature when the patient looks down (Fig. 14).

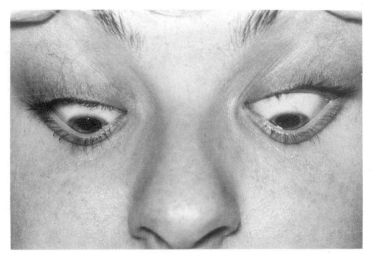

Fig. 14 Keratoconus (note contact lens on right eye)

Corneal dystrophies

This is an obscure group of conditions of unknown cause. Occurring more commonly in adult life and with a familial tendency, corneal opacities develop and interfere increasingly with vision. Both eyes are affected: there are no inflammatory signs, except in rare superficial dystrophies in which there may be recurrent epithelial erosion. The pathological progress cannot be reversed by medical treatment, but corneal grafting usually gives improvement if necessary.

Fuchs' dystrophy is of particular importance in the elderly. It is a degenerative condition which affects the endothelium, with a tendency to corneal oedema when the endothelial cells are no longer numerous or healthy enough to maintain corneal clarity. When associated with cataract it presents a difficult problem for the surgeon, who is faced with the need to carry out both cataract extraction and full-thickness corneal grafting. Fuchs' dystrophy may recur after grafting.

Congenital limbal dermoid

This congenital, non-progressive tumour occurs at the limbus and covers a variable extent of the cornea. It is pearly-white, elevated, and may have hairs in its surface. Excision is normally required on cosmetic grounds, though a permanent scar remains at the site of the tumour.

TRAUMATIC CONDITIONS

Corneal abrasion

This is an injury to the cornea which goes no deeper than the epithelium: the possible causes are numerous. There is intense pain, with lacrimation, photophobia and blepharospasm. The diagnosis is confirmed by staining the cornea with fluorescein (Plate 13) (see p. 2). Examination is easier if the eye is anaesthetised with a drop of local anaesthetic, and if there is the possibility of a foreign body, a thorough search of the conjunctival sac, with eversion of the upper lid (see p. 28) is necessary.

Treatment is with antibiotic ointment and a firmly applied pad until the epithelial defect has healed: normally within 24–48 hours. Infection and failure to heal will lead to corneal ulceration.

Recurrent corneal erosion

Apparently trivial corneal injuries may lead to intermittent recurrence of symptoms over a long period. After the initial abrasion has healed, the patient wakes with intense pain in the morning because an area of unstable epithelium has been stripped off by the upper lid on opening the eye. The pain and photophobia subside later in the day, as adjacent corneal epithelial cells slide over and cover the defect. The condition may result from any injury: a mother whose eye is injured by her baby's finger is typical.

Treatment. It is helpful to refer these cases for examination with a slit lamp. Plentiful application of ointment at night for a month or two is usually effective. Any eye ointment which does not contain steroids will do, but hypertonic saline in ointment form, if available, is considered most helpful. Alternative treatments are the removal of the affected area of epithelium with alcohol, after anaesthetising the cornea, or the use of a soft, 'bandage' contact lens for an extended period.

Welder's flash ('arc eye')

Welder's flash and snow blindness are similar conditions due to exposure to ultraviolet light. After an interval of 6 or 8 hours, intense bilateral lacrimation, blepharospasm and photophobia develop. The patient may only have been a spectator.

Examination is impossible until the eyes have been anaesthetised with 1% amethocaine. Once the blepharospasm has been relieved and the cornea stained with fluorescein, multiple punctate erosions are seen. The lesions heal within a few hours. Local anaesthetic and reassurance are the only treatment required.

Foreign bodies

Usually there is a clear history of the source of the foreign body. Other irritants, such as misplaced or loose eye lashes or a subtarsal foreign body, may give rise to discomfort and cause the patient to suspect there is something in the eye. A good light and magnification help with removal. A drop of local anaesthetic such as 1% amethocaine is instilled and the foreign body removed. If the foreign body is loosely adherent to the cornea it may be removed with a cotton wool 'bud' or the corner of a tissue. A sterile 17-gauge needle is a convenient instrument to pick a foreign body off the cornea. Antibiotic ointment should be given four times a day for 4 days after removal of a corneal foreign body and the patient asked to report back if the eye is not comfortable, or if vision is blurred. Mydriatics are usually unnecessary: atropine, with its prolonged effect, is never required. After a metallic foreign body, a rust ring is very often found: it is more readily removed after 2 or 3 days' use of antibiotic ointment. This may more easily be done in a specialist department.

Prevention is better than cure, and patients should be advised about protective measures.

Perforations of the cornea

All perforations, and cases in which there is the slightest suspicion, should be referred immediately and the patient instructed to take nothing by mouth in order to be suitable for general anaesthesia.

A history of hammering metal on metal with no evident superficial foreign body suggests an intra-ocular metallic fragment, and the finding of a subconjunctival haemorrhage heightens suspicion. X-ray examination of the eye usually demonstrates a metallic foreign body, however small.

Laceration of the cornea may lead to shallowing of the anterior chamber compared with the fellow eye, or distortion of the pupil. Injury to deeper structures may be seen as lens opacities or haemorrhage within the eye (see p. 90).

Early detection is of great importance in successful management. Damage to ocular structures by a retained intra-ocular foreign body, or by infection or resulting retinal detachment may be irreversible. 'Missed' intraocular foreign bodies are an unfortunate but regular cause of justified medico-legal claims. If there is any suspicion of penetration, refer to hospital.

CORNEAL INFLAMMATION (Keratitis)

A corneal ulcer is any breach in the corneal epithelium other than a traumatic abrasion. It is usually painful. The history may reveal previous episodes of corneal ulceration or other eye disease, or suggest the possibility of a foreign body or trauma. Systemic disease such as rheumatoid arthritis should also be noted.

There will be reduced visual acuity if the central portion of the cornea is involved. Fluorescein staining and inspection with a good light and magnification will show the size, situation and shape of any ulcer. Further examination may indicate lid abnormalities or dry eye (see p. 25).

If contact lenses are worn they should be suspected as the cause of any keratitis.

Causes of corneal ulceration

Bacterial infection
Viral infection
Fungal infection
Exposure or foreign body
Toxic reaction

Bacterial corneal ulcer

Infection usually enters the cornea after the epithelium has been breached by minor injury. The eye is painful, photophobic and waters. The patient complains of a sensation of something in the eye, due to movement of the lids over the epithelial defect.

The eye is red, most markedly in the quadrant where the ulcer lies. Visual acuity is usually reduced, especially if the centre of the cornea is involved. A greyish area of oedema and opacity may be seen before stain is used. Fluorescein demarcates the edges of the ulcer. A search should be made for a foreign body on the cornea, in the fornices of the conjunctival sac or under the upper lid.

Treatment is with antibiotic ointment and a firm pad. More severe inflammation may require the addition of 1% atropine drops twice daily to dilate the pupil and reduce vascular engorgement in the anterior segment of the eye, as any severe corneal lesion is associated with some degree of iritis.

If treatment of a corneal ulcer does not produce a cure in 3 or 4 days the patient should be referred.

Hypopyon keratitis

A severe corneal ulcer may produce so extensive an iritis that cellular debris settles to produce a level of pus — *hypopyon*. Any patient with a hypopyon ulcer should be referred: full bacteriological study and oral and intensive topical antibiotic treatment will be needed.

Marginal keratitis (Fig. 15)

This represents a local hypersensitivity reaction to conjunctival infection by certain organisms — usually *Staph. aureus.* Conjunctivitis may be slight, but there is photophobia, pain and vascular congestion at the limbus. Round or elongated ulcers or sub-epithelial corneal infiltrates may be seen within the limbus. These do not progress centrally. In addition to treating the conjunctivitis with antibiotic drops or ointment, a topical steroid may be used. This is one of the few situations where the use of combined antibiotic-steroid preparations is justified in a short course, *provided dendritic ulcer is not present.*

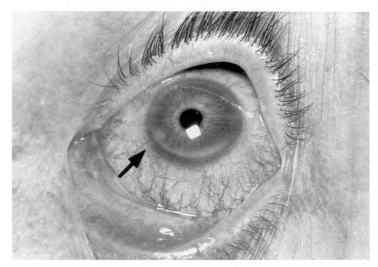

Fig. 15 Marginal keratitis (arrowed).

Viral keratitis

Herpes simplex keratitis (dendritic ulcer)

Herpes simplex keratitis is initially confined to the corneal epithe-lium. Primary infection is seldom recognised in the eye, but the secondary dendritic ulcer is a common and serious condition. It presents as an irritable eye and is diagnosed after fluorescein stain-ing (Plate 14) as a branching ulcer.

Treatment is with any of a number of anti-viral ointments:

Idoxuridine (Kerecid, Stoxil, Ophthalmidine)
Vidarabine (Vira-A)
Acyclovir (Zovirax)

The ointment should be used five times daily until the ulcer has healed: drops should be used hourly. Padding is usually unnecess-ary. Owing to the problems which may arise from herpes simplex keratitis it is advisable to refer all patients, but treatment may be started by the general practitioner as soon as the diagnosis is made. Recurrence is common, and should be treated in the same way. Steroid preparations should never be used in general practice if herpes simplex infection is suspected.

Complications. Amoeboid ulceration is a more advanced form in which the ulcer spreads to assume a confluent pattern. Treatment is with anti-viral agents.

Disciform keratitis and kerato-uveitis. Herpes simplex infection of the deeper layers of the cornea leads to central corneal thickening and opacification described as 'disciform keratitis'. There is usually associated uveitis and treatment is difficult and needs to be carefully monitored in a specialist unit; frequently, *diluted* steroid drops are used at the same time as an anti-viral agent. It may take months until the inflammation settles. Permanent scarring of the cornea is common and may necessitate corneal grafting.

Fortunately herpes simplex keratitis usually affects only one eye.

Herpes zoster (Fig. 16)

Corneal ulceration may occur during the acute stage of ophthalmic herpes zoster: conjunctival inflammation, uveitis and secondary glaucoma are also seen. A dendritic-like ulcer may occur. In the later stages corneal sensation may be impaired and lid deformities occur, resulting in chronic keratitis which is difficult to manage.

Treatment. This is controversial. Acyclovir (Zovirax) ointment five times daily to the affected eye during the acute stage has been shown to reduce the incidence of ocular complications. It may be difficult to

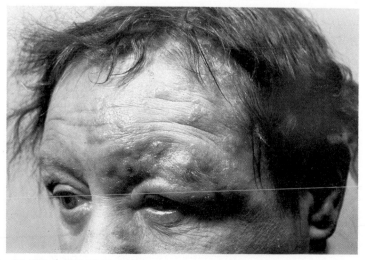

Fig. 16 Ophthalmic herpes zoster

open the lids, but a relative or nurse should be able to get some ointment into the conjunctival sac. Vesicles on the nose suggest eye involvement: when in doubt, it is better to give than to withhold treatment. Oedema of the lids of the uninvolved eye commonly occurs.

Treatment of the skin eruption is equally controversial. Idoxuridine solutions (Herpid or Iduridin) and acyclovir (Zovirax) cream are reputed to be effective if applied for about four days early in the illness. These antiviral agents are principally active in herpes simplex; they are expensive and of disputed value in zoster. Alternatives are a steroid cream or an anti-infective agent such as 10 per cent povidone iodine (Betadine) cream or paint.

Systemic treatment is a logical approach as the virus is in the affected nerves. Oral acyclovir (Zovirax) is currently under clinical trial, but is not yet of proven value.

Admission to hospital should be considered for any case in which the eye is involved. The advice of an eye specialist should be sought if the eye cannot be adequately examined by the general practitioner, or if it is significantly inflamed or the vision impaired.

If the patient is not admitted to hospital, analgesics will be required and maybe a systemic antibiotic if there is secondary bacterial infection.

Adenoviral keratitis

This epidemic condition is discussed under conjunctival infections (p. 32).

Fungal keratitis

Injuries, particularly by vegetable matter, occasionally cause corneal ulcers which are resistant to conventional antibiotic treatment. Necrotic material seen in the ulcer bed may prove to contain fungi.

In common with other corneal ulcers which fail to respond to antibiotics, referral is essential.

Other forms of keratitis

Kerato-conjunctivitis sicca

The triad of dry eyes, dry mouth and collagen disease particularly affects patients with rheumatoid arthritis. The symptoms are discomfort and sometimes mucoid discharge, occasionally progressing to frank corneal ulceration with severe pain. Staining with *rose bengal* (obtainable in solution as Minims) shows multiple small red dots on cornea and conjunctiva, representing epithelial defects. Defective tear production may be confirmed by Schirmer's test (see p. 25). Dry eyes are common in older people without systemic disease.

Treatment is with artificial tear supplements, of which numerous preparations are available. They should be used for symptomatic relief as often as the patient requires them. Dry eye is a variable condition and the need for drops will change according to the patient's state as well as the prevailing atmospheric conditions. Dry environments such as centrally heated houses with inadequate humidification and cars with the heaters blowing hot air are particularly troublesome.

Severe cases should be referred for assessment by an ophthalmologist: surgical occlusion of the lacrimal puncta may be a helpful additional measure, and mucolytic drops such as acetylcysteine 5 or 10% may also be recommended.

Other rheumatoid complications. Any rheumatoid patient with painful eyes not responding to artificial tear supplements should be referred for slit lamp examination of the eye and further assessment.

Neuroparalytic keratitis

Loss of corneal sensation deprives the cornea of one of its protective mechanisms and ulceration frequently follows. Apart from herpes zoster affecting the ophthalmic division (see p. 51) any lesion of the fifth nerve producing corneal anaesthesia may lead to keratitis. Protection of the cornea by the copious use of ointment at night and spectacles with protective side pieces may be sufficient. Patients at risk of corneal ulceration should be referred: tarsorrhaphy (temporary or permanent partial closure of the lids), or 'bandage' soft contact lenses may be required.

Rosacea keratitis (Plate 15)

Rosacea is a chronic disorder involving the face — reddening of the skin, telangiectasia and episodes of inflammation. The cause is unknown. Ophthalmic complications are blepharitis, chalazia, conjunctivitis and keratitis.

Corneal involvement begins as marginal vascular infiltration: ulceration and opacification may follow. Treatment with low dosage (250 mg b.d.) oral tetracycline for at least 2 months usually controls exacerbations. The tablets should be taken between, not with, meals.

Bell's palsy

Idiopathic facial palsy may lead to corneal ulceration from exposure. While waiting for the facial nerve to recover it is important to supply the patient with plenty of antibiotic ointment to put in the affected eye at night. If this proves inadequate, the patient should be referred for temporary lateral tarsorrhaphy.

Dysthyroid exophthalmos

Proptosis due to this or any other cause may place the cornea at risk owing to exposure. Dysthyroid eye disease is considered further on page 130, but the same principles apply. Plenty of ointment at night is the first measure.

Other causes of exposure keratitis

Any severe debilitating disease may lead to the patient sleeping with imperfectly closed eyes, with consequent drying and ulceration of the cornea, seen as a lack of normal lustre in the epithelium. Ointment should be instilled regularly. In severe cases, padding of the eyes with a paraffin gauze square under the pad may be necessary until normal lid closure is re-established.

DEGENERATIVE CONDITIONS OF THE CORNEA

Band-shaped opacity

In some degenerate eyes and in those which have sustained previous injury or ulceration, a horizontal band opacity develops in the interpalpebral portion of the cornea, associated with the deposition of calcium in its superficial layers. Patients with this condition should be referred — treatment with chelating agents applied under local anaesthesia may be considered worthwhile.

Pterygium

A degenerative condition arising in the conjunctiva and extending horizontally as a wing-like opacity of the cornea (see p. 34).

MATERIAL FOR CORNEAL GRAFTING

Techniques for storing donor corneal material in tissue culture have been developed, but many eye departments use only fresh donor material for grafting. Occasionally an eye is removed for other reasons (such as intra-ocular tumour) which has a healthy cornea suitable for grafting, but most material is obtained from cadavers. The eye — or just the cornea with a surrounding ring of sclera — must be removed within 6 hours of death and stored at 4° C.

If a patient who has expressed the wish to be a corneal donor dies at home, the general practitioner should contact the nearest Eye Department as soon as possible after death and arrangements will be made for the corneae or eyes to be collected.

Most often the corneae are taken from patients who die in hospital, with the consent of the relatives if no donor card was carried.

7

The middle coat of the eye

ANATOMY

The vascular, pigmented middle coat of the eye, known as the uveal tract, consists of three parts — iris, ciliary body and choroid. The iris diaphragm lies against the lens, separating the anterior and posterior chambers. The ciliary body produces aqueous humour and, by its attachment to the lens by zonular fibres, controls accommodation through the action of the ciliary muscle (parasympathetic, third nerve).

The sphincter pupillae (parasympathetic, third nerve) and dilator pupillae (cervical sympathetic) control the size of the pupil. The highly vascular choroid and the central retinal artery together nourish the retina.

CONGENITAL ABNORMALITIES

Aniridia

The iris is absent.

Albinism

Pigment is absent from the eye (ocular albinism) or from the whole body. Vision is poor and nystagmus occurs. Albinoid children should be referred for specialist assessment.

Colobomata (Fig. 17)

Incomplete closure of the foetal choroidal fissure of the developing eye leaves a defect in the uveal tract in its lower nasal quadrant. Colobomata extending posteriorly in the choroid may be associated with poor vision.

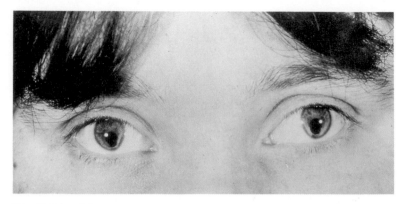

Fig. 17 Iris colobomata

TRAUMA

Non-perforating eye injuries due to squash balls, shuttlecocks, etc, small enough to enter the orbit may damage the uveal tissues.

Hyphaema (Plate 16)

Bleeding into the anterior chamber causes blurred vision. When the blood has time to settle, a level is seen in the anterior chamber. Patients with hyphaema are usually referred to hospital because of the possibility of secondary haemorrhage: though uncommon, this can be disastrous. Contusion severe enough to produce hyphaema frequently causes damage to the anterior chamber angle and may lead to glaucoma years later (p. 121).

If a patient with traumatic hyphaema cannot be admitted to hospital, bed rest should be advised until the blood has been absorbed.

Traumatic mydriasis

Paralysis of the iris sphincter following a contusion injury: recovery is usual.

Iridodialysis

A tear of the iris root.

Choroidal tear

Force from a contusion injury transmitted to the posterior segment of the eye may result in a crescentic tear of the choroid, usually temporal to the disc. Severe visual impairment may result; there is no treatment.

UVEAL INFLAMMATION

Suppurative inflammation of the uveal tract is usually obvious and requires urgent referral. *Non-suppurative* uveitis, an important cause of blindness, is more difficult to diagnose and remains poorly understood.

Although occasionally secondary to other ocular disorders such as keratitis and cataract, most cases of uveitis are endogenous.

Acute anterior uveitis (iritis) (Plate 17)

This is the form which is of greatest concern to the general practitioner. Presenting as a red and painful eye, there is engorgement of the ciliary vessels around the limbus; the pupil is usually small and may be irregular, adhering to the lens (posterior synechiae). Visual acuity is frequently impaired. Clumps of leucocytes adhering to the posterior surface of the cornea (keratic precipitates) may be seen under magnification. Keratic precipitates and posterior synechiae are diagnostic of uveitis. Exact diagnosis can be difficult and requires a slit lamp for confirmation. All suspected cases should be referred urgently.

The *cause* in most cases cannot be found although more than half have the HLA B27 antigen. Systemic disorders such as juvenile rheumatoid arthritis, sarcoidosis, ankylosing spondylitis and Reiter's disease may be found.

Treatment is with topical corticosteroids and atropine or other drugs to dilate the pupil. Steroids administered systemically or by injection around the eye are required if drops fail to control the inflammation. Recurrences are common. A patient known previously to have uveitis who presents again to his general practitioner may be treated initially with steroid drops provided examination of the cornea with fluorescein has shown no dendritic ulcer to be present.

Ciliary body inflammation (cyclitis)

Inflammation presenting in childhood or adolescence in one or both eyes with gradually deteriorating vision, associated with opacities in the anterior vitreous, is known as *pars planitis*. Steroid treatment may be recommended, but the condition is relatively benign. Specialist follow-up is necessary.

Posterior uveitis (choroiditis, chorio-retinitis)

This condition is painless and the eye is usually white. Blurred vision or a chance finding of fundus lesions at routine ophthalmoscopic examination are the usual modes of presentation.

Most cases are of unknown cause and treatment is correspondingly haphazard and unrewarding. Systemic granulomatous conditions such as sarcoidosis, tuberculosis and syphilis are occasionally found.

Two specific forms of posterior uveitis deserve mention:

1. Toxoplasmosis

Either a congenital or acquired infection. The former is of significance in the eye, but the acquired disease, which may occur at any age, usually causes no symptoms. The organism, *Toxoplasma gondii* is ingested either from partly-cooked, infected meat or from soil contaminated with animal faeces containing the cysts of the parasite. The domestic cat is probably the animal reservoir. If a pregnant woman becomes infected the organisms reach the foetus through the placenta, leading to congenital toxoplasmosis.

Congenital toxoplasmosis (Plate 18). The organism has a predilection for central nervous tissue and, in the extreme form, causes severe brain damage. Convulsions may be the first symptom. Ocular toxoplasmosis produces scarring in the retina and choroid — a white lesion surrounded by accumulated black pigment in the inactive stage. Such a focus at the posterior pole prevents development of macular vision.

Toxoplasmosis lesions in the eye may undergo apparently spontaneous reactivation, producing signs of posterior uveitis, often with associated inflammation in the anterior segment. Cloudiness of the vitreous causes blurred vision: visual loss is profound if the reactivated focus lies near the macula or optic disc.

Diagnosis is usually made on clinical grounds, but antibody tests such as the toxoplasmosis dye titre may help. The test is positive at low titres in many individuals without affected eyes, and the titre seldom changes during an exacerbation of ocular inflammation.

Treatment is unnecessary unless vision is impaired, but any patient known to have ocular toxoplasmosis who notices blurred vision should be referred. Steroids by mouth or intra-orbital injection, combined with drugs active against the organism, usually sulphonamides, pyrimethamine (Daraprim) or tetracycline are usually prescribed.

2. Toxocariasis

Infection of the eye by the nematode worm *Toxocara canis* is an uncommon but serious form of posterior uveitis, usually occurring in young children who play in ground contaminated by the excrement of puppies which have not been 'wormed'. The parasite reaches the posterior pole of the eye, producing a choroido-retinal lesion which irreversibly destroys central vision. Fortunately, it is generally unilateral. Presentation usually results from routine visual acuity testing or the detection of a squint. There is no useful treatment.

TUMOURS OF THE UVEAL TRACT

Iris

Tumours of the iris are rare, but any patient concerned that a tumour may be developing should be referred for a specialist opinion.

Ciliary body

Malignant melanoma rarely develops in the ciliary body causing distortion of the pupil or detachment of the retina. These tumours, if not too large, may be treated by local resection with preservation of useful vision.

Choroid

Benign melanoma

Flat, pigmented areas usually occur in the posterior half of the fundus. They are seldom significantly elevated and there is no associated retinal detachment. Distinction between larger benign melanomata and malignant tumours may be difficult — cases of doubt should be referred for observation and serial fundus photography unless the patient's life expectancy from other causes does not warrant long-term follow-up.

Malignant melanoma

These life-threatening tumours arise anywhere in the fundus. The lesion is elevated and tends to cause an associated retinal detachment, with peripheral visual field loss and, later, impairment of central vision. Intra-ocular enlargement leads to secondary uveitis and glaucoma, and eventually the tumour may perforate the sclera and invade the orbit directly. Distant metastases are common. Any suspected malignant melanoma of the choroid should be referred.

Treatment is controversial: patients treated by enucleation have been shown to be at greater risk of dying from metastases in the years immediately following surgery than those left untreated. Conversely, the prospect of extra-scleral extension cannot be viewed with equanimity. Local resection with preservation of the eye is sometimes feasible. Patients over 70 are probably best untreated unless the tumour is large.

Metastatic tumours (Plate 19)

These tumours present similarly to malignant melanoma, but their growth is more rapid. Palliative radiation may be justifiable. Tumours arising from breast carcinoma usually respond to Tamoxifen.

8

Cataract

Any opacity in the lens is a cataract. The term should be used carefully in the presence of patients as it still conveys visions of a painful operation, a long period of partial blindness and uncertain cure. Many cataracts are non-progressive or develop slowly, and it is only a small proportion that needs treatment by the surgeon.

CLASSIFICATION OF CATARACT

1. Congenital cataract.
2. Cataract associated with other disorders:
   a. metabolic disorders
   b. syndromes of multiple congenital deformity
   c. skin disorders
   d. drugs
   e. physical causes: trauma, heat, ionising radiation
   f. secondary to other eye disease.
3. Senile cataract.

Congenital cataract

The lens is an ectodermal structure developed by the infolding of a vesicle from the surface ectoderm. Within this vesicle layers of lens fibres are developed, the oldest being forced towards the centre and the youngest fibres being found on the surface. Many types of opacity develop as a result of interference with normal development of the lens. Only a few lead to visual symptoms and these may sometimes be traced to a definite upset in maternal health during pregnancy. Rubella, in particular, contracted by the mother during the first trimester of pregnancy conveys a definite risk of the child being born with congenital defects in the eye, ear or heart. Cataract due to rubella is a sporadic disorder: many congenital cataracts are familial.

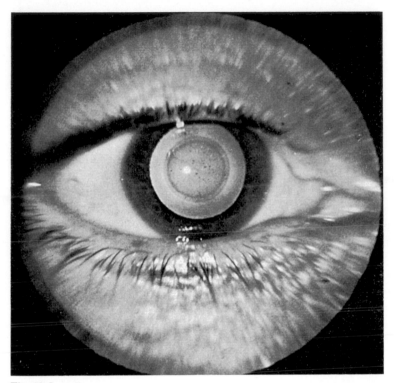

Fig. 18 Lamellar cataract

Congenital cataract may be unilateral or bilateral, complete or incomplete. Incomplete cataracts, in which the fibres being laid down at the time of an illness are opaque and the remainder of the lens clear are known as *lamellar* (*zonular*) *cataracts* (Fig. 18). While the majority of congenital lens opacities do not increase after birth, some types, particularly of a punctate variety, become more dense in later life and may then require surgical attention.

Indications for treatment of congenital cataract

Dense cataracts present from birth are detected by ophthalmoscopic examination: attention may be drawn to them by lack of visual awareness in the child. If bilateral, these cataracts demand urgent referral if useful visual results are to be obtained. They are rare.

In the child the need for treatment depends purely upon the density of the opacity. If a child is able to benefit from normal schooling there is probably no need to interfere, for removal of a lens leads to destruction of the eye's power of accommodation with its consequent disabilities. Operation may sometimes be requested in a unilateral case if the opacity is so dense as to produce a white appearance in the pupil.

If it is decided that treatment is indicated, surgical removal of the lens is usually successful and holds out the only hope of producing useful vision. The early onset of visual defect and the presence of associated nystagmus often make the ultimate visual result disappointing.

Surgical treatment of congenital cataract is usually by aspiration, leaving the posterior capsule intact. This may subsequently become opaque and a discission or 'needling' restores vision again. Lensectomy, with removal of the entire lens and part of the anterior vitreous is an alternative technique. On clearance of the pupil a corrective lens must be provided to replace the lost refractive power of the eye, either by a convex spectacle lens or by a contact lens which, in infants, is of the soft or hydrophilic type suitable for wear for extended periods. Hard contact lenses may be used by older children. The use of intra-ocular lenses in children is still controversial. Restoration of binocular vision is seldom achieved in young children after surgical treatment of unilateral congenital cataract.

After such operations, delayed complications, particularly detachment of the retina, are not uncommon.

Cataract associated with other disorders

Metabolic disorders

1. *Diabetes mellitus.* Temporary cataracts lasting a few weeks as a complication of diabetes are very rare. However diabetics tend to develop senile cataract at an earlier age than non-diabetics, and it is standard practice to test the urine of new patients presenting to an eye clinic with a diagnosis of cataract. In one study 3% were found to have diabetes, previously undiagnosed. The management of cataracts does not differ from non-diabetics but post-operative complications are rather more common and removal of a dense cataract may reveal diabetic retinal changes.

2. *Galactosaemia.* Cataracts in newborn infants with galactosaemia are reversible if appropriate treatment is given early.

3. *Hypocalcaemia.* Cataract may follow hypocalcaemia from any cause — characteristically of the sub-capsular type at the anterior and posterior poles of the lens.

4. *Dystrophia myotonica*. Significant visual impairment by cataract is usual by the age of 40.

Syndromes of multiple congenital deformity

In Down's syndrome, characteristic cataracts tend to become apparent about puberty.

Skin disorders

Cataract is associated with certain diseases of the skin — atopic dermatitis for example.

Drugs

Steroids given over long periods, topically or systemically, may cause cataract formation — typically of the posterior sub-capsular type which interferes markedly with vision.

Physical causes: trauma, heat, ionising radiation

1. *Trauma*. Injury to the lens capsule leads to opacification of the fibres of the lens due to their exposure to aqueous. A small hole in the capsule may lead to a limited opacity, but more extensive injury leads to the rapid opacification of the entire lens, which may swell, causing secondary glaucoma.

Contusion, without rupture of the lens may lead to a characteristic rosette-like cataract, which may also progress rapidly to total opacity.

Treatment depends on the age of the patient, any associated injury and the state of the fellow eye. Surgery is usually indicated and is most commonly done by the extracapsular method. Optical correction of the resulting aphakia may be provided either by a contact lens or an implant to restore binocular vision.

2. *Radiation*. Infra-red, microwave and ionising radiation may cause cataract.

Secondary to other eye diseases

Longstanding eye disorders such as chronic uveitis and persistent retinal detachment commonly lead to cataract.

Senile cataract

This is the most important group. Senile cataract is usually bilateral, though the opacity in one lens may be more advanced than the other.

Symptoms

The patient complains of visual deterioration. Apparently sudden deterioration may sometimes be due to longstanding unilateral cataract which has suddenly come to the patient's attention. The rate of progress of cataract is variable, but some morphological types interfere with vision more rapidly than others.

Cataracts of the nuclear sclerosis type, causing increase of refractive index in the nucleus of the lens, present with increasing myopia. Such patients may, having required a presbyopic spectacle correction for reading, enjoy a period in which they can read unaided.

Diagnosis

The diagnosis is made by examination of the eye with an ophthalmoscope through a dilated pupil. A cataract is most easily seen from a distance of about 30 cm with a +5 lens in the ophthalmoscope: the red reflex in the pupil is broken by opacities within the lens.

Treatment

The only effective treatment of senile cataract is surgery. This is indicated if the opacity is causing visual impairment sufficient to interfere with the patient's normal occupation and recreation despite accurate correction of any refractive error and provision of adequate lighting. The mere existence of a cataract in one or both eyes is not itself an indication for surgery. Hypermaturity of a cataract may make operation essential to avoid complications due to the cataract — lens-induced glaucoma and uveitis.

Selection of patients for surgery

No patient need be considered too old or frail for cataract surgery. The pre-operative assessment includes examination of the anterior and posterior segment of the eye to detect other conditions which might predispose to complications — for example, corneal dystrophy — or prejudice the result of uncomplicated surgery — for example, macular degeneration. A decision must be made about the patient's suitability for general or local anaesthesia.

Optical correction of the aphakic eye

The need for optical correction of the aphakic (lens-absent) eye determines policy in every case. Removal of the lens renders the eye markedly hypermetropic and correction of this defect by a spectacle lens gives a difference in retinal image size between the operated and unoperated eyes of about 30%. This cannot be tolerated if the fellow eye retains clear vision: *spectacle* correction of aphakia is therefore inappropriate after surgery for unilateral cataract with a normal fellow eye.

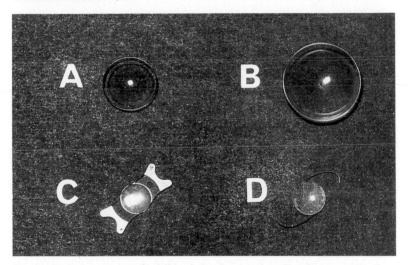

Fig. 19 Optical correction of aphakia: A, hard contact lens; B, soft contact lens; C, anterior chamber implant (Choyce type); D, posterior chamber implant (Sinskey type)

Contact lenses and *intra-ocular lens implants* (Fig. 19) provide the possibility of both eyes being used when only one has been subjected to cataract surgery. *Contact lenses* may be of the 'hard' type suitable for daily wear, or 'soft' or hydrophilic lenses, suitable for either daily or extended wear (see p. 99).

Lens implants are becoming increasingly popular, both with patients and surgeons. They are fixed in the eye in one of three ways:

supported by the sclera in the anterior chamber, attached to the iris, or placed in the posterior chamber within the residual lens capsule after extracapsular cataract extraction. All three methods give good results, and their selection is largely a matter of the surgeon's preference. Once in situ, the lens implant may be forgotten, whereas contact lenses require handling and, in many cases, long-term medical supervision of the patient.

The use of contact and intra-ocular lenses makes it possible to offer cataract surgery whether one or both eyes are affected, though many surgeons have reservations about the use of implants in younger patients.

Techniques of cataract surgery

A detailed discussion of techniques is not proposed, but there are three methods of surgical removal of cataract:

1. *Intracapsular extraction*, in which the lens is removed entirely within its capsule, either by forceps or cryoprobe. This is the most commonly used method, but it is unsafe in children and young adults owing to adhesion between the lens and vitreous.

2. *Extracapsular extraction*, in which the anterior capsule of the lens is removed, the nucleus expressed and residual cortical material aspirated from the eye. The posterior capsule is left intact. This may become thickened leading to impaired vision in the months or years post-operatively. Capsulotomy, an out-patient procedure, restores vision.

3. *Phako-emulsification*, a modification of the extracapsular method, whereby the lens nucleus is fragmented by a probe oscillating at ultrasonic frequency and simultaneously aspirated from the eye. Its advantage is that a 3 mm incision suffices and the patient is thereby more quickly rehabilitated: the long-term results do not differ from the other two methods. The equipment for phako-emulsification is expensive.

All three methods give excellent results and are suitable for either local anaesthesia with basal sedation, or general anaesthesia. The extracapsular method has become more popular recently owing to the introduction of capsule-supported lens implants. A period of 6–8 weeks must elapse before the prescription of definitive glasses after surgery owing to post-operative refractive changes — this period coincides with the need of most patients for post-operative drops. If a patient is confused after cataract surgery and is using long-acting mydriatic drops such as atropine or hyoscine, these may be the cause. The drops should be stopped and the ophthalmologist informed.

After glasses have been dispensed out-patient supervision can usually be discontinued.

9

The retina and vitreous

ANATOMY

The retina develops as an outgrowth of the fore-brain and is invaginated to form two layers. The outer becomes the retinal pigment epithelium and the inner, the sensory retina, with the rods and cones adjacent to the pigment epithelium and the nerve fibre layer innermost.

The posterior segment of the globe is filled by transparent vitreous gel with a collagenous fibrillary structure. Passing across the vitreous is the embryonic hyaloid vessel system. With ageing, and particularly in myopic eyes, the vitreous undergoes liquefactive changes (synersis). In the elderly the posterior surface of the vitreous commonly becomes detached from the retina and optic disc, and the hyaloid remnants are visible to both patient and observer as a large 'floater'.

The blood supply of the retina is from the central retinal artery, except at the macula where the tissues are supplied by diffusion from the innermost layer of the choroid — the chorio-capillaris. The central retinal artery divides into four main branches, each accompanied by a tributary of the central retinal vein. The diameter of each vein exceeds that of the corresponding artery in a 3:2 ratio. Where they cross there is, in the normal fundus, no interference with the direction of either vessel.

ARTERIOSCLEROTIC AND HYPERTENSIVE RETINOPATHY

Arteriosclerosis is seen in the retinal vessel walls (Plate 20). Sclerotic changes are most obvious at arterio-venous crossings: the arterial walls lose their transparency and obscure the view of the underlying vein on either side of the column of blood. More severe arteriosclerosis leads to increasing pallor of the arterial light reflexes and

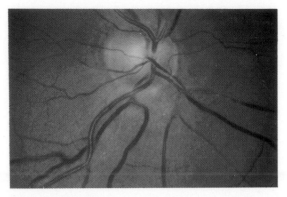

Plate 20 Retinal arteriosclerosis

more marked crossing changes, with greater tortuosity of the larger vessels and a change of direction at the crossing from the normal oblique angle towards a right angle. The vein distal to the crossing may be distended.

Advanced arteriosclerosis is seen as marked pallor of the arterial light reflex and irregularity of the lumen, with yellowish sheathing of the vessel walls, like the stem of a clay pipe. The blood column may disappear completely in places. In extreme cases the vessels may appear to be entirely occluded, though their patency can be shown by fluorescein angiography.

HYPERTENSION (Plate 21)

Younger patients with severe hypertension show narrowing of the arterioles. Prolonged hypertension leads to structural changes in the vessel walls, the hypertrophied smooth muscle becoming replaced by fibrous tissue.

Older patients in whom there is significant arteriosclerosis show arterio-venous crossing changes and irregularity of arteriolar calibre. More severe and longstanding hypertension may result in further retinal changes — haemorrhages, 'hard' exudates, retinal infarcts (cotton wool spots, or 'soft' exudates) and disc oedema.

Retinal haemorrhages in hypertension are most commonly seen in the superficial, nerve fibre layer of the retina. They may be linear or flame-shaped and are most numerous near the optic disc. Haemorrhages confined to one sector of the fundus signify localised retinal vascular occlusion (see p. 76). Haemorrhages seldom interfere with vision unless one occurs at the macula.

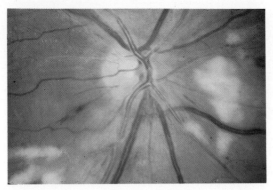

Plate 21 Hypertension (haemorrhages and 'cotton wool' spots)

'Hard' exudates are yellowish-white deposits in the deeper layers of the retina. They represent accumulated fat deposits and the residue of oedema. Their size varies from small dots to areas greater than the diameter of the disc. They are commonly found in the region between disc and macula and in a star-formation around the macula.

'Cotton wool' spots are retinal infarcts in the nerve fibre layer: they are accumulations of degenerate axoplasm. The term 'soft' exudate has largely been abandoned to avoid confusion with 'hard' exudates. Cotton wool spots occur in the most severe forms of hypertensive retinopathy and therefore indicate a grave prognosis. They are also seen in other systemic disorders — for example, diabetes (see p. 82), collagen disorders, blood dyscrasias and the acquired immune deficiency syndrome ('AIDS').

Optic disc oedema

Since the classification of hypertensive retinopathy by Keith, Wagener and Barker (1939), this has been regarded as the surest indicator of malignant hypertension. However, cotton wool spots invariably accompany disc oedema and they, too, justify the placing of a hypertensive patient in this category. The co-existence of other features of hypertensive retinopathy and the slight elevation of the optic disc help differentiate this condition from papilloedema due to raised intracranial pressure (see p. 126).

RETINAL VASCULAR OCCLUSION

Central retinal artery occlusion

Failure of the retinal circulation leads to sudden and profound visual loss. If the occlusion persists, the ischaemic retina sustains irreversible damage, with swelling of the inner retinal layers due to accumulation of degenerate axoplasm. Usually occurring in the elderly, central retinal artery occlusion may be due to an embolus from the carotid or to thrombosis of an already arteriosclerotic vessel.

The presenting symptom is sudden, painless loss of vision in one eye. Examination shows the absence of direct pupillary light reaction (see p. 7) and pale, attenuated retinal vessels (Plate 22). With

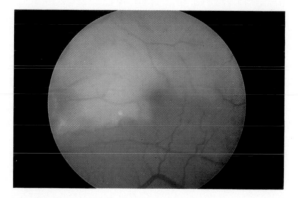

Plate 22 Retinal artery occlusion, superior branch

progressive retinal damage, generalised retinal oedema is seen, except at the macula. Here the retina is thinnest and the area appears as a reddish spot owing to visibility of the underlying choroidal circulation.

Unless the occlusion was caused by an embolus which passed into a more peripheral vessel, relieving the central obstruction, visual loss is permanent and optic atrophy becomes apparent after a few weeks. The retinal oedema subsides. There may be an audible carotid bruit.

Table 8 shows the various tests required in the investigation of central retinal artery occlusion.

Table 8 Investigation of central retinal artery occlusion

General	Blood
Urinalysis	Blood count, ESR/plasma viscosity
Blood pressure	Plasma lipids
ECG	
(Carotid angiography)	

Management in the first few minutes consists of attempting to lower intra-ocular pressure to encourage the onward passage of any embolus. *Firm massage* of the globe through the closed lids is the most effective treatment available to the general practitioner. The patient should be referred for ophthalmological assessment and review of the carotid arteries and cardiovascular system.

Retinal branch arterial occlusion

Also presenting as sudden, painless loss of vision, the portion of the visual field lost depends upon the extent of retinal arterial closure.

Amaurosis fugax

Transient occlusion of the central retinal artery or one of its branches gives rise to 'fleeting blindness'. The patient usually complains of a 'curtain' obscuring vision for a few minutes. This is a form of transient ischaemic attack and is often the precursor of a major cerebrovascular accident. An embolus may be visible in one of the retinal arterioles. Giant cell arteritis (p. 123) is a less common cause: the diagnosis depends on finding a raised ESR.

A carotid bruit should be sought. The only certain way to demonstrate significant carotid stenosis in the absence of a bruit is by carotid angiography — only indicated in patients in whom endarterectomy would be considered. Aspirin 300 mg daily is often recommended to reduce the likelihood of further transient ischaemic episodes, although its effectiveness is controversial.

Central retinal vein occlusion

Occlusion of the central vein has a less dramatic presentation than that of the artery, owing to the variable element of ischaemia that accompanies venous obstruction. Visual loss is usually profound,

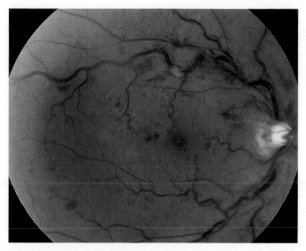

Plate 23 Incomplete central retinal vein occlusion:
predominantly superior temporal branch

developing over a period of hours or days. Occasionally the visual defect is only slight. The fundus appearance (plate 23) is typically dramatic, with extensive haemorrhages throughout, often as if red paint had been thrown at the retina; there may be numerous 'cotton wool' spots. Secondary glaucoma may occur about 3 months later (p. 122).

Aetiology

Central retinal vein occlusion is predominantly a disease of the elderly. More than 60% have high blood pressure, and generalised cardiovascular disease and diabetes are also commonly found. Raised intra-ocular pressure, with or without established open angle glaucoma, is also an important aetiological factor. Haematological abnormalites such as dysproteinaemias and blood dyscrasias should be excluded. Oral contraceptives may be a contributory cause.

Every case should be referred for ophthalmological assessment as well as medical screening.

Eventually the haemorrhages and 'cotton wool' spots clear, but the retina is usually damaged irreversibly, with loss of central vision due to ischaemia and macular oedema. The most helpful factors in the patient's management are the correction of hypertension and other treatable circulatory and biochemical abnormalities.

Retinal branch vein occlusion

Occlusion of part of the retinal venous circulation occurs more commonly than central vein occlusion, and usually affects one of the branches on the temporal side. Occlusion is distal to a crossing point and the haemorrhages and 'cotton wool' spots are confined to the affected sector of the fundus. If the macula is involved, central vision will be affected; otherwise the condition may pass unnoticed by the patient and be found at a routine fundus examination.

The aetiology is the same as that of central vein occlusion and the patient should be similarly referred for investigation.

Vitreous haemorrhage

The symptoms of vitreous haemorrhage vary from the appearance of a few spots before the eye to sudden and complete painless visual loss. The diagnosis is made by finding blood in the vitreous on examination with a 'plus' lens in the ophthalmoscope — or by being able to see nothing at all with the instrument if the haemorrhage is severe and the vitreous totally opaque.

Vitreous and other intra-ocular haemorrhages may occur spontaneously in perfectly healthy people, especially on severe exertion or the performance of a Valsalva manoeuvre. Trauma is also an important cause; but apparently spontaneous vitreous haemorrhage requires urgent referral in case there are other abnormalities within the eye.

Diabetes, hypertension and blood dyscrasias must be excluded and the patient investigated to identify treatable vascular disease (Table 8). Full fundus examination should be carried out by an ophthalmologist at the earliest opportunity. If retinal details cannot be seen satisfactorily, the patient is kept under periodic review until, with the clearance of the haemorrhage, a view of the fundus is obtained.

A number of retinal disorders may present with haemorrhage into the vitreous — a retinal tear or detachment, retinal vein occlusion or localised vascular abnormality. New vessel formation associated with vein occlusion, diabetes, sickle cell disease or retinal vasculitis may be found. Their diagnosis is a matter for the ophthalmologist.

Persistent vitreous haemorrhage may be treated surgically, by vitrectomy.

MACULAR DEGENERATION

This profoundly affects central vision while sparing peripheral, 'navigating' vision. It is the commonest reason for blind registration in developed countries. A disorder of old age, pigmentary abnormalities, haemorrhages and oedema are seen at the posterior pole. Rarely, macular degeneration occurs in younger patients as an inherited disorder. With few exceptions, it cannot be treated.

High myopia is frequently associated with macular degeneration in which the choroid and retina become progressively atrophic at the posterior pole leaving extensive areas of white sclera exposed to view with the ophthalmoscope. The fundus of a myopic eye is most easily seen if the patient wears his spectacles or contact lens.

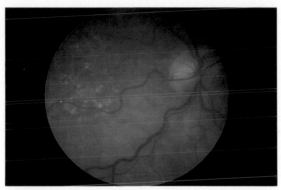

Plate 24 Senile macular degeneration (age 75). Right eye: Colloid bodies and pigment atrophy. Vision: 6/9.

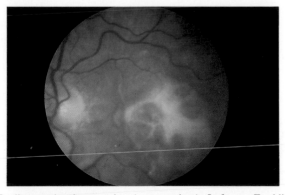

Plate 25 Senile macular degeneration (same patient). Left eye: Established disciform macular degeneration. Vision: Hand movements.

Senile disciform macular degeneration is a common form of macular degeneration to which increasing attention has recently been directed owing to the possibility of offering treatment to a few patients (Plates 24 & 25).

Predisposed eyes show yellowish spots (colloid bodies) in the membrane beneath the retina. New vessels arise from the choroid and grow forwards beneath the retina. Unlike normal retinal vessels, fluid leaks from these abnormal capillaries and the retina becomes elevated at the posterior pole causing disturbance of vision. Distortion, abnormal colour vision and a slight drop in acuity are the first symptoms.

If the condition is diagnosed at an early stage, when the new vessels do not extend beneath the fovea and there is no sub-retinal haemorrhage, it may be possible to destroy the abnormal vessels by laser and prevent further fluid accumulation. If the condition is not diagnosed at this stage and treated successfully, an organised haemorrhage develops beneath the macula and central vision is irreversibly destroyed. Even apparently successful treatment may be followed by a further episode of new vessel formation and fluid leakage: there is no cure for ageing.

The interval between the earliest symptoms and irreversible changes is about 2 weeks, so disciform macular degeneration is most unlikely to be diagnosed in time for treatment in the first eye. However it is a strongly bilateral condition and any patient known to have lost central vision in one eye who subsequently develops symptoms of visual blurring or distortion in the other should, if possible, be referred urgently in case anything can be done.

Patients with bilateral macular degeneration usually maintain a fairly high level of independence provided they are given appropriate advice and support. For further discussion of blind and partially-sighted registration, see page 137.

DRUG TOXICITY IN THE RETINA

Retinal damage may result from the prolonged administration of certain drugs — particularly chloroquine and some phenothiazines.

Quinine may cause rapid bilateral visual loss. Recovery in a few days is usual.

DIABETIC RETINOPATHY

The exact cause of diabetic retinopathy is not known but experimental and clinical evidence shows that it is in part related to diabetic control. Never seen at the onset in young diabetics, retinopathy has an increasing incidence the longer the duration of diabetes. The elderly, maturity-onset diabetic may present with retinopathy or its complications before other symptoms of diabetes occur.

Classification

The object of any classification of diabetic retinopathy is to indicate:

a. the present extent of retinopathy
b. the need for treatment
c. the likely prognosis.

The underlying abnormality is in the walls of small vessels in the retina and this leads to local formation of micro-aneurysms, vessel leakage, exudation and capillary closure. Retinal ischaemia following capillary closure results in new vessel formation. Sight is damaged by oedema, exudation at the macula, haemorrhage arising from damaged and abnormal vessels and retinal detachment caused by fibrosis of new vessels and traction on the retina.

Management of diabetic retinopathy

Although prevention of retinopathy may be impossible, good control must always be the aim in managing diabetic patients. Laser or photo-coagulation is now widely available in eye departments and its introduction has fundamentally changed the management of diabetic retinopathy and made vigilant observation essential. Diabetics who are pregnant need to be watched with particular care.

All diabetic patients, except juvenile onset diabetics with disease of less than 10 years duration, should have an annual retinal examination after testing visual acuity and dilating the pupils of both eyes with a short-acting mydriatic (e.g. tropicamide (Mydriacyl) 0.5%).

Any doctor taking responsibility for the care of diabetic patients should ensure that this requirement is fulfilled. If significant retinopathy is found the interval should be reduced to 6 months. Any cases in whom there is doubt about the need for laser treatment should be referred for further assessment. Early treatment is far more effective than late. It is little use waiting for the patient to lose central vision in one eye before referring. Hypertensive and ischaemic changes may complicate diabetic retinopathy: again, if in doubt, refer. The categories shown in Figure 20 are considered below:

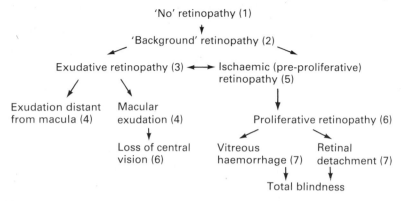

Fig. 20 Classification of diabetic retinopathy (the numbers refer to the paragraphs in the text

1. *'No' retinopathy*. The normal appearance of the fundi in diabetes is a safe indication that no retinal treatment is needed — at least until next year's follow-up! But fluorescein angiography of apparently normal eyes frequently shows extensive changes not visible by ophthalmoscopy — so there is little cause for complacency. Angiography is not necessary routinely.

2. *'Background' retinopathy* (Plate 26). The earliest visible changes in diabetic retinopathy are micro-aneurysms and haemor-

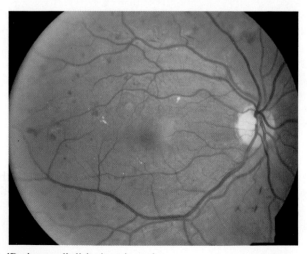

Plate 26 'Background' diabetic retinopathy

rhages. Micro-aneurysms appear as tiny red dots. The haemor-rhages are characteristically of the 'dot' and 'blot' type which lie in the deeper layers of the retina. Hard exudates are also seen, though if they appear near the macula the classification of the fundus should be 'exudative' retinopathy and the patient referred. 'Background' retinopathy should be followed up every 6 months by the doctor managing the patient's diabetes.

3. *Exudative retinopathy* (Plate 27). Significant 'hard' exudates constitute grounds for referral, particularly if they are near the macula. Typically, exudates accumulate in rings around a central area of micro-vascular leakage. Treatment of this area with laser coagulation usually causes the exudation to regress. Retinal tissue damaged by hard exudates does not recover its function, even though the exudation may disappear; hence the need for treatment before the onset of visual impairment. Macular oedema may be difficult to detect in the absence of hard exudates. Vision is impaired.

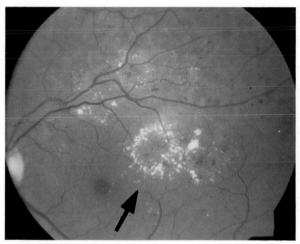

Plate 27 'Exudative' diabetic retinopathy

4. *Advanced exudative retinopathy*. Irreversible damage to the macula results in permanent loss of central vision. The patient becomes eligible for blind registration if both eyes are affected, as in advanced senile macular degeneration, but useful 'navigating' vision is maintained. Regular observation is still required in case the retina develops features of proliferative retinopathy (see 5–7).

5. *Ischaemic (pre-proliferative) retinopathy* (Plate 28). The signs of impending new-vessel formation in the retina — and later the iris

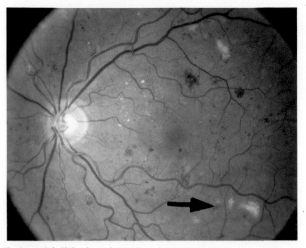

Plate 28 'Ischaemic' diabetic retinopathy. Arrow indicates cotton wool spots

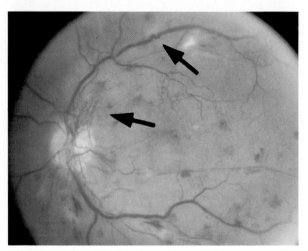

Plate 29 'Proliferative' diabetic retinopathy. Arrows indicate new vessels and a venous loop

and anterior chamber (rubeosis iridis) with its disastrous consequences — are those of ischaemia of the tissues. 'Cotton wool' spots
(retinal infarcts) are the cardinal sign, with distension of the veins
into sausage-like segments and the formation of loops. Any suspicion of these changes or of the appearance of new-vessel networks
either on the optic disc or peripherally demands urgent referral for
laser treatment (see 6).

Treatment usually consists of the application of multiple laser burns (3000 or more) to the retinal periphery. By reducing the metabolic requirements of the retina as a whole, this removes the stimulus to new-vessel formation so that already-developed new vessels regress and no more appear. The treatment is an out-patient procedure, often given in several sessions. Follow-up is likely to be carried out in the ophthalmic clinic after laser treatment.

6. *Proliferative retinopathy* (Plate 29). New vessels, initially in the plane of the retina and subsequently growing forwards into the vitreous, are seen on the optic disc or elsewhere in the fundus. Their appearance indicates urgent need for referral and laser treatment. Failure to treat the retinopathy adequately at this stage leads inexorably to loss of vision (see 7).

7. *End-stage proliferative retinopathy*. Vitreous and subhyaloid haemorrhage and retinal detachment are disasters requiring referral. The usual practice with vitreous haemorrhage is to wait for it to clear spontaneously. If it does not, and the ophthalmologist considers that the state of the underlying retina justifies surgery, the blood may be cleared by vitrectomy and the retina treated by photocoagulation from within the eye. Both this and the surgical treatment of diabetic traction retinal detachment by vitrectomy techniques are 'last-ditch' procedures. Blindness resulting from proliferative retinopathy is, unlike the exudative type, usually complete.

Until more satisfactory metabolic management of diabetes prevents retinopathy — and the other vascular complications elsewhere in the body — regular, informed review of the fundi and referral for laser treatment as described above are the doctor's essential duty to his diabetic patients.

RETINOPATHY OF PREMATURITY (Retrolental fibroplasia)

Now a rare condition, retinopathy of prematurity reached epidemic proportions in the 1940s, before its cause was understood. In common with proliferative diabetic retinopathy, abnormal new vessels grow forwards from the retina in response to ischaemia.

The administration of oxygen to premature babies with respiratory distress, resulting in high arterial Po_2, causes retinal vasoconstriction: if maintained, this becomes irreversible in 3–4 weeks. On reducing the oxygen concentration of the baby's environment, proliferative changes occur in the retinal circulation.

Infants thought to be at risk should be examined by an eye

specialist. The peak incidence of abnormal retinal vessel formation and fibrosis is about 7 weeks after full term. Mild cases usually show regression of the proliferative fibro-vascular tissue thereafter, but more severe cases develop myopia and permanent retinal changes. Since the recognition of the cause, progression to retinal detachment and blindness are no longer seen.

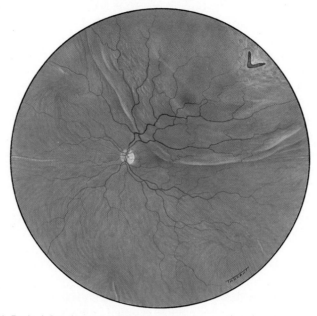

Plate 30 Retinal detachment with retinal break

RETINAL DETACHMENT (Plate 30)

A common treatable cause of blindness, retinal detachment is of importance to the general practitioner because he may be consulted by patients with early symptoms when prompt referral and treatment are all-important. He must therefore recognise the symptoms and signs.

The condition is mis-named. The detachment is of the sensory retina (rods and cones) from the underlying pigment epithelium, with fluid accumulation in the potential space between these parts of the retina — inaccurately termed 'sub-retinal' fluid. Detachment is usually associated with one or more breaks in the sensory retina.

Diagnosis

Predisposing factors are myopia, particularly in the middle-aged, previous trauma, cataract surgery and a family history of retinal detachment. There is a strong bilateral tendency, so any retinal breaks or detachment in the fellow eye are also relevant.

Warning symptoms are *flashing lights* in the eye, associated with increased *floaters*, and *spots* before the eye. Retinal detachment causes a *visual field defect* corresponding to the area detached. The patient may complain of a 'curtain' across the visual field. Any patient presenting with these symptoms should be sent for urgent examination by an eye surgeon even if no retinal detachment is seen. 'Spots' before the eye may signify a small vitreous haemorrhage if a retinal break passes across a blood vessel. When examined through a dilated pupil, the detached retina appears greyish-blue and may be ballooned forward into the vitreous, the vessels appearing blacker than those on the normal, attached retina.

The diagnostic problem in patients with symptoms suggestive of retinal detachment but no central visual loss is to distinguish 'innocent' degenerative vitreous changes from retinal breaks or early retinal detachment. At the ophthalmologist's disposal are more effective techniques for examining the peripheral retina — sometimes a very difficult task — and this responsibility should be passed on by the general practitioner.

Management

The retinal breaks are located and sealed by cryotherapy and other surgical means. Provided the macula is not detached at the start of treatment, excellent restoration of vision is usually possible. Established macular detachment inevitably leads to some permanent impairment of function. Detachment of the superior retina, threatening to involve the macula, demands the most urgent surgical attention and the patient should lie flat until this can be achieved. The patient should be able to return to work about 6 weeks after retinal detachment surgery, but 'contact' sports and knocks on the head should be avoided indefinitely.

RETINAL DETACHMENT WITHOUT A RETINAL BREAK

Intra-ocular tumours, particularly malignant melanoma, may produce retinal detachment below the tumour. The detachment is likely to be the presenting feature by causing loss of vision, the tumour having previously been unnoticed.

Exudative, serous detachment may also occur in systemic disorders such as renal failure and ocular inflammatory disorders such as scleritis.

ECLIPSE BURN OF THE RETINA

Rarely occurring now, ill-advised observation of an eclipse of the sun produces a macular burn sufficient to reduce central visual acuity permanently. Careless handling of a laser may cause a similar disaster.

INHERITED DISORDERS OF THE RETINA

Retinitis pigmentosa (Plate 31)

Retinitis pigmentosa is the commonest of a group of disorders, often with systemic associations, presenting with night blindness and progressive visual field loss.

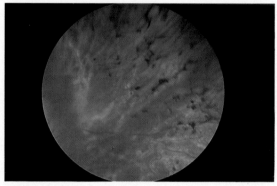

Plate 31 Retinitis pigmentosa: note 'bone corpuscle' pigment clumping and attenuation of vessels

Inheritance

Retinitis pigmentosa may be transmitted as an autosomal dominant, recessive or X-linked recessive. About 50% of cases arise with no previous family history: most are probably autosomal recessive.

Presentation

Night blindness is the first symptom, usually appearing in childhood. The more severe cases — typically with recessive inheritance — become aware of visual field loss in the second decade, and fundus changes are visible. Progressive field loss makes these patients blind by the fourth or fifth decade, although less severe forms of the disease may not interfere with vision until old age. Cataract may be a complicating factor.

Diagnosis

The fundus appearance is characteristic, with 'bone corpuscle' pigment clumping, particularly in the mid-periphery of the retina, attenuation of the retinal vessels and waxy pallor of the optic disc. Special testing of dark adaptation and of the electrical function of the retina enable a diagnosis to be made in cases of doubt.

Management

No treatment is effective, but patients may be helped by suitable counselling, retraining and aids for partially sighted or blind. Contact with the Retinitis Pigmentosa Society may be of comfort to many patients, and genetic counselling should be made available to those who request it. Patients with retinitis pigmentosa should not drive.

TUMOURS OF THE RETINA

Retinoblastoma is a rare and potentially lethal malignant tumour which may arise by spontaneous mutation or be inherited as an autosomal dominant. The diagnosis is usually made in the first 6 months of life by the appearance of a white mass in the pupil or a squint. Although conservative treatment may be possible, enucleation of the affected eye is usually necessary unless the diagnosis is made when the tumour is small.

Regular follow-up for the first 5 years is essential for the early detection and treatment of tumours arising in the fellow eye: about 30% are bilateral.

Any child with persistent squint or a white mass in the pupil should be referred, the latter urgently.

INFLAMMATORY DISORDERS OF THE RETINA

These are considered in Chapter 7.

10

Trauma

BLUNT INJURY

Without rupture of the globe

Such injuries are caused by fists, blows during sport, and a multitude of domestic and industrial mishaps. The effects range from a simple 'black eye' to gross disorganisation of the globe.

The cornea may be abraded (see p. 46). Conjunctival lacerations merit referral because of the possibility of concealed rupture of the globe. They may require suturing.

There may be sub-conjunctival haemorrhage from rupture of conjunctival blood vessels but, provided vision is unimpaired, this needs no treatment.

Bleeding into the anterior chamber shows as diffuse haziness of the aqueous, obscuring details of the iris and of the deeper parts of the eye. The blood settles to the lowest part where it lies with a characteristic fluid level (see Plate 16). Sometimes the anterior chamber becomes filled with blood, a condition which may lead to secondary glaucoma. Admission to hospital is advised.

There may be dilatation of the pupil (mydriasis). This usually recovers spontaneously. Alternatively the root of the iris may be torn (irido-dialysis).

Traumatic cataract sometimes follows contusion to the eye: its appearance can be delayed. In severe injuries, the lens may be torn from its attachment to the ciliary body (subluxation or dislocation) prolapsing forward through the pupil or falling back into the vitreous. The finding of gross visual defect will point to injury of this kind.

In the posterior segment of the eye, there may be bleeding into the vitreous or damage to the retina. Retinal oedema (commotio retinae) shows as a greyish area in the fundus where detail is obscured and there may be small retinal haemorrhages. Commotio retinae resolves with rest. It is occasionally followed by pigmentary retinal changes and permanent visual loss. The retina may be torn by the distortion of the eye at the time of the injury, leading to retinal detachment and increasing visual failure. This may be delayed for months or years. Treatment is surgical. (see p. 84).

Choroidal tears are sometimes seen and appear as scars, concentric with the optic disc and close to the posterior pole. These represent areas of choroidal atrophy through which the sclera is visible.

Rupture of the globe

Sometimes the coats of the eye are not able to resist the pressure at the moment of impact and rupture occurs, most commonly at the junction of cornea and sclera. There will be haemorrhage within the eye. Examination will show the rupture and there will usually be ocular contents presenting in the wound. Vision is grossly impaired and these injuries are unlikely to be missed unless lid swelling prevents adequate examination. Some attempt must always be made to examine the eye and to assess visual acuity. Defective vision, as in any eye problem, is the finding most likely to indicate the possibility of serious trouble.

PENETRATING INJURIES

Without retention of a foreign body

Potential causes include scissors, bows and arrows, darts, flying particles, particularly in industry, and windscreens.

The resultant injury is usually severe, though penetration by such things as fine wire can be difficult to see.

There will be a history of something having struck the eye; the eye will be photophobic and watering and the vision impaired. If the wound is in the anterior part of the eye, the pupil is usually distorted and there may be prolapse of iris through the wound. Examination of the deeper eye is difficult on account of photophobia and haziness of the ocular structures. The lens may become opaque.

In a child, examination of an injured eye is particularly difficult. A child is sometimes loath to admit that he has sustained an injury. It may not be until the eye becomes red and painful during the subsequent days that the true condition is apparent.

Treatment of these wounds is surgical, with wound toilet and repair. The prognosis for vision must be guarded.

With retention of a foreign body

These injuries are almost always industrial. The commonest cause is the hammer, striking a chisel or other metal tool. This may throw off a flake of steel which penetrates the eye. Although provided with goggles, workers often fail to protect themselves adequately. Travelling at high speed, these flakes of steel are usually sterile and enter the eye through a small wound. The worker may scarcely notice the incident, subsequently complaining simply that he got 'something in his eye'. This makes diagnosis difficult and those dealing with men engaged in the type of work described should be constantly aware of the possibility of a penetrating injury, if the foreign body is not visibly embedded in the surface of the cornea.

A piece of steel in the eye will, in the course of months or years, induce a chronic chemical reaction and will ultimately destroy sight. This is known as *siderosis bulbi*.

Examination may show a wound of entry, perhaps with prolapse of iris, and this is not likely to be mistaken. Difficulty arises if the

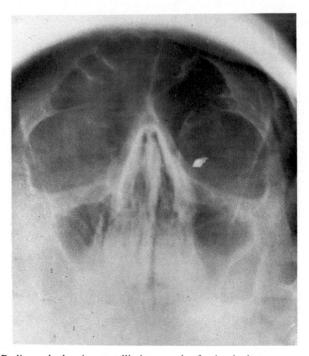

Fig. 21 Radiograph showing metallic intra-ocular foreign body

entry wound is small, perhaps lying at the margin of the cornea, or in the sclera where it is covered by conjunctiva. A localised subconjunctival haemorrhage is a danger signal.

The cornea must be stained with fluorescein and the eye examined in a good light. Even if the entry wound is not visible, a hole in the substance of the iris is diagnostic of a foreign body retained within the eye.

The only sure diagnosis is by X-ray (Fig. 21) and this should be routine in any case where the presence of an intra-ocular foreign body is suspected.

Treatment involves repair of the wound and removal of the foreign body after X-ray localisation. Removal is by magnet if the particle is of steel.

Sympathetic ophthalmia

This rare condition may follow a penetrating injury of the eye. Persistent inflammation in the injured eye may lead to low-grade iridocyclitis in the fellow eye after 2 or 3 weeks. This can be very destructive and difficult to control. The cause of the condition is poorly understood, but it represents a sensitivity reaction in the second eye. The decision whether or not to remove an injured eye is, therefore, always an anxious one.

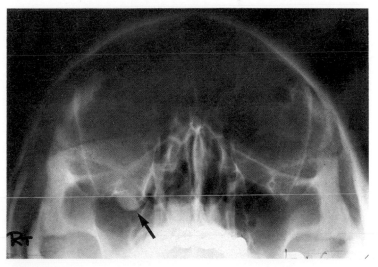

Fig. 22 Radiograph of blow-out fracture of orbit: note 'tear drop' opacity in antrum

INJURIES TO THE ORBIT

Orbital haematoma may follow contusion, and fracture of the orbital bones may displace or damage the extra-ocular muscles.

Double vision suggests the possibility of a *'blow-out' fracture* (Plate 32) and all contusion injuries leading to double vision should be referred. In 'blow-out' fracture an extra-ocular muscle becomes trapped in a fracture of the floor, or occasionally the medial wall of the orbit. There is enophthalmos, due to prolapse of the orbital contents, and limitation of movement, usually on upward gaze.

The X-ray finding of a 'tear-drop' opacity in the antrum (Fig. 22) is characteristic of a 'blow-out' fracture of the orbital floor. The orbit may have to be explored to free the trapped muscle and cover the bony defect.

Occasionally a blow to the head may interfere with the delicate blood supply of the optic nerve as it passes through the optic canal, causing severe visual impairment in the affected eye. Optic nerve damage is indicated by an afferent pupillary defect (p. 7). Optic atrophy appears after a few weeks. There is no effective treatment. A squint, usually divergent, may develop later.

11

Spectacles and contact lenses

The similarity between the eye and the camera is well known. The formation of a clearly focused image depends on the presence of a normal relationship between the axial length of the eye and the focal length of the lens system.

The term 'lens system' is used to indicate that there are two elements involved in the refraction of light entering the eye. One is the biconvex lens and the other, more powerful from the optical point of view, the convex anterior surface of the cornea.

Accommodation

If the eye is to obtain a clear image of objects at varying distances, there must be a mechanism to adapt the focal length of the lens system to suit the varying angle of the entering rays. This is done by alteration in the curvature of the lens of the eye.

Consisting of a transparent mass of lens matter enclosed in an elastic membrane (the lens capsule), the lens is suspended within the circle of the ciliary body by a series of fine fibres (the zonule or suspensory ligament).

The ciliary body contains a mass of muscle fibres innervated by the parasympathetic element of the third cranial nerve and is able, by its contraction, to alter the tension in the suspensory ligament and thus in the lens capsule. Contraction of the ciliary muscle increases the curvature of the lens and so shortens its focal length. This focuses the eye for near objects.

The stimulus for accommodation is reflex, based on the need to maintain a clear retinal image (Fig. 23). There is a natural relationship between the accommodative effort required to produce a clear retinal image and the amount of convergence of the visual axes to keep the images on the maculae of both eyes. The importance of the balance between these two functions is considered in the discussion of errors of refraction in relation to the aetiology of squint (Fig. 27, p. 104).

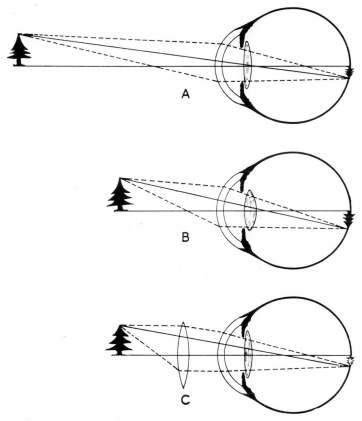

Fig. 23 Formation of the retinal image. (A) In the normal eye, with the accommodation relaxed, the image of a distant object falls on the retina. (B) When the object approaches the eye a change of shape of the lens takes place and the image remains focused on the retina. This is accommodation. (C) With increasing age the eye loses its power to change its focus for close objects and has to be reinforced by convex lenses to keep the image in focus. This is presbyopia.

Presbyopia

As age increases, the lens of the eye becomes larger and less able to respond to the efforts of the ciliary body to alter its curvature. At the age of about 45 reading and sewing become more difficult, and at about 65 all power of accommodation is lost.

There is no evidence that 'resting' the eyes or the performance of any so-called 'exercises' have any influence on the development of presbyopia or of any other eye condition. The middle-aged must simply accept the need to wear glasses for close work. Whether these be reading glasses, bifocals, or 'half-moons' is purely a matter of choice.

Hypermetropia (long sight)

This is the commonest refractive error. Almost universal in infants, it becomes less in the growing years.

In hypermetropia, the accommodation being relaxed, rays of light from an object in the distance are brought to a focus behind the retina (Fig. 24). In youth, if the degree of hypermetropia is slight, this defect is no disadvantage as it can be overcome by accommodation — but reading may be an effort (see p. 133).

Hypermetropia needs correction only if it is of such a degree as not to be comfortably overcome by the use of the eye's own focusing mechanism. Exceptions are children with convergent squint or with amblyopia of one eye due to unequal refractive errors (p. 109).

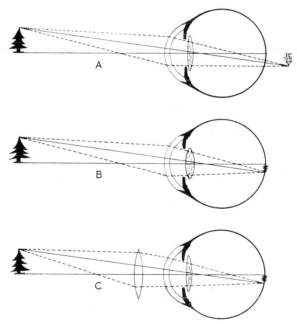

Fig. 24 Hypermetropia. (A) With the accommodation relaxed, the image of a distant object falls behind the retina. (B) An effort of accommodation is required for the clear viewing of an object, even in the distance. (C) This effort has to be increased as the object becomes closer. If the error cannot comfortably be overcome by accommodation, a convex spectacle will be needed.

A degree of hypermetropia insufficient to cause symptoms in youth may, with the natural lessening of the power of accommodation, give rise to reading difficulties in middle life. There will be an earlier demand for reading glasses than in the patient with no refractive error (the emmetrope).

Myopia (short sight)

In myopia, rays of light from a distant object are focused in front of the retina (Fig. 25): the myope is at a disadvantage compared to the hypermetrope in that he is unable to obtain clear distant vision by the exercise of his accommodation. At close distances, however, the advantage is with the myope, who can focus on near objects with little or no effort of accommodation.

Myopia is of two types: simple myopia, which is common, and progressive, or degenerative myopia, which is uncommon.

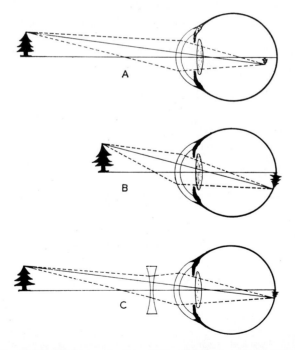

Fig. 25 Myopia. (A) The image of a distant object falls in front of the retina and any effort of accommodation will only increase the blurring. (B) Near objects, on the other hand, are seen clearly with little or no accommodation. (C) For clear distant sight, concave glasses are needed.

Simple myopia

Simple myopia has a strong hereditary tendency. With growth, the globe becomes too long. The onset is usually about puberty, hence the term 'school short-sight'; but it may be delayed into early adult life.

The system of routine examination of school children generally leads to prompt recognition of the condition, or the teacher notices that the child is not reading the blackboard from the back of the class. In pre-school children, parents complain that a child holds books very close to his face or sits too near the television.

Simple myopia advances during the school years and the need for new glasses can only be determined by regular examination. The child can then lead a normal life and can play most games — in splinterproof glasses or contact lenses. It is not essential that he wears his glasses from morning to night, as he probably will not take kindly to the idea of glasses in any case; but they should be worn in class and at other times when clear distant vision is required. As he grows older, he will decide for himself when glasses are to be worn.

Particular attention should be paid to the vision of siblings when there is a short-sighted child in the family.

Measures to slow or arrest the progress of myopia have been tried: the latest is radial keratotomy in which incisions are made in the periphery of the cornea. Neither this nor any other 'treatment' of myopia has gained general acceptance.

Degenerative myopia

A condition of unknown cause associated with very high degrees of refractive error and with pathological changes within the eye. Among these are vitreous opacities, cataract formation and degenerative changes at the posterior pole of the eye, often leading to destruction of central vision.

Retinal detachment is more common in myopes than in normally-sighted individuals, the incidence increasing with the degree of myopia.

Astigmatism

This may be associated with either hypermetropia or myopia, the term astigmatism implying that the curvature of the cornea is not symmetrical in all meridia. It requires a cylindrical lens for its correction. Failure to correct higher degrees of astigmatism in the years of visual development may lead to partial amblyopia.

There are some pathological conditions which, by causing distortion of the cornea, produce irregular astigmatism. Among these are diseases of the cornea such as keratoconus, corneal ulceration of various types, and the results of injury.

In irregular and severe astigmatism the refractive error may not be corrected by ordinary spectacles, and the provision of a contact lens may be the solution.

Ocular headache

In the lay mind, the occurrence of headache is so often blamed on the need for glasses that it seems appropriate to mention the subject here.

Headache is a very common complaint, and it is certainly prominent among the reasons for which patients are referred for an ophthalmic opinion. There are some features of headache which may point to the eyes being implicated in a given case.

The ocular headache is usually related to, or precipitated by, use of the eyes. Thus it occurs on prolonged reading or sewing, watching television, or taking up a clerical occupation for the first time. It is usually relieved by ocular rest. The pain may be delayed in onset, appearing in the morning after an evening of ocular activity. It may be felt in the eyes themselves, or in the temple or occiput, in which case it is probably coming from the neck muscles.

Ocular headache is usually regular in occurrence. A pain appearing at long intervals, without any change of ocular habit, is not likely to be of ocular origin. The same can be said of a pain of recent onset, without there having been any change in the use of the eyes.

Sufferers from *migraine* often present with ocular symptoms — flickering lights, hemianopia, and so on; but the headache which follows is unlikely to be influenced by the provision of glasses.

Refractive changes in diabetes

About a third of diabetics, particularly those with higher levels of blood glucose, show a temporary change of refraction towards myopia at the onset of the illness. This can precede other symptoms by several weeks or months. Patients in the presbyopic age group may find their reading glasses unnecessary but their distance vision blurred. An unexpected myopic shift in refraction should suggest the possibility of diabetes and the urine be tested for glucose.

Transient hypermetropia frequently occurs as the blood sugar level falls on starting treatment: glasses should not be prescribed until the condition has been stable for several weeks.

Contact lenses

Contact lenses may be used as an alternative to spectacles for the correction of all refractive errors. In general, the higher the refractive error, the greater the benefit of contact lenses. But their use on cosmetic grounds and on account of the unobstructed vision they provide constitute important reasons for many patients' preference for contact lenses instead of spectacles. Occasionally contact lenses are ordered as part of the treatment of eye disorders rather than on purely optical grounds, for example, in keratoconus where the astigmatism is too irregular to be corrected by spectacles, and in some cases of corneal ulceration, for protective purposes.

Contact lenses are of two main types, according to the material from which they are made: hard and soft (hydrophilic).

Hard lenses

Hard contact lenses are most commonly made of perspex. This material is inexpensive, durable and easily worked. Its major disadvantage is the barrier it constitutes to diffusion of oxygen into the cornea. Deprivation of oxygen leads to corneal thickening owing to fluid retention, and oedema of the corneal epithelium causing discomfort and blurred vision.

Hard contact lenses have to be fitted so as to minimise oxygen deprivation and, in general, their wear must be restricted so that the oxygen supply to the cornea can be replenished between periods of wear. Greater oxygen transmission can be achieved with hard lenses by drilling small holes in them — fenestration. To overcome this problem, other 'hard' contact lens materials have been developed, with greater oxygen transmission than perspex. These are the so-called 'gas-permeable' hard lenses. They have some disadvantages compared with perspex on the grounds of cost, fragility and the tendency to attract protein deposits.

Problems. The commonest problems presented by wearers of hard contact lenses to the doctor are associated with oxygen deprivation, usually caused by wearing the lenses too long, and minor trauma resulting from their insertion or removal. Patients with problems associated with hard lens wear should be advised not to use the lens for 48 hours. The wearing time should then be extended gradually, as most patients are advised when beginning to use hard lenses.

An apparently lost contact lens may sometimes be found in the superior conjunctival fornix on everting the upper lid (see p. 28).

Women taking oral contraceptives may have slightly impaired tolerance of contact lens wear.

Soft lenses

Soft, or hydrophilic, lenses are made from a variety of materials which conform to the curvature of the cornea and have the property of allowing gas diffusion. Lenses made from these materials are larger than hard lenses — usually they overlap the corneal margin by 1 to 2 mm — and they must at all times be kept in a fully hydrated state. If the lenses are allowed to dry they shrink and become brittle and cannot be used until re-hydrated.

The advantages of soft lenses are longer initial wearing times and greater initial comfort — though wearers who become accustomed to hard lenses usually find them eventually just as comfortable as soft lenses. Many soft lens materials allow extended wear for days, weeks or even months. Others, with lower gas permeability, are suitable only for daily wear and must be removed before the wearer goes to sleep.

Problems. Sterility is of great importance with soft contact lenses as the water-permeable material may become contaminated by bacteria. Care has to be taken when handling the lenses and most patients use chemical or thermal disinfection. It is with these chemicals, usually chlorhexidine and thiomersal, that the most frequently encountered problems with soft lenses are associated. The disinfecting chemicals are toxic in high doses and accumulate in the contact lens. The *symptoms* of toxic effects of lens disinfectants are lens intolerance and discomfort. The *signs* (Plate 33) are red eye, with hyperaemia and follicle formation, and hypertrophy of conjunctival papillae. A soft lens wearer who becomes intolerant of disinfecting chemicals is usually advised to change to boiling the lenses in normal saline without preservative.

Infection, with corneal ulceration, is a less common but serious problem. Ulceration can lead to corneal vascularisation. Should this occur, soft lens wear must be discontinued until the ulcer has healed and all new vessels have regressed. Antibiotic drops are prescribed. Gradually increasing corneal vascularisation may also occur without infection — probably in response to hypoxia.

Soft lenses give less satisfactory visual acuity than hard lenses if used to correct refractive errors which include significant degrees of astigmatism. They are also less durable than hard lenses and have to be discarded if damaged, discoloured or affected by protein deposition.

Technique for removal of a contact lens (Fig. 26, overleaf.)

A general practitioner may occasionally be called upon to remove a contact lens from an eye which is, for any reason, irritable or inflamed. For example, the elderly aphakic patient who had been fitted with an extended wear soft lens who is unable to get to the specialist:
1. Open the eye widely with the index fingers behind the lashes of each lid.
2. Gently press the lid margins together so that they touch the edges of the contact lens. This will release the lens from the surface of the eye. The lens can then be picked off the lid margin.
3. If the first attempt is not successful, try again.

Tear production

Inadequate tear secretion is often a cause of poor tolerance of contact lenses of any type. This can be assessed by Schirmer's test (p. 25).

Drugs and contact lenses

Printed on the packets of some eye drop preparations are the words: 'not to be used with contact lenses'. This is a controversial matter, and it applies only to soft lenses — never to hard. There are two possible reasons for advising against the use of certain eye drops with contact lenses:
1. Because the drops may, in the long term, damage or discolour the contact lens.
2. Because the drops contain a preservative — commonly benzalkonium chloride — to which the lens wearer may develop a local adverse reaction.

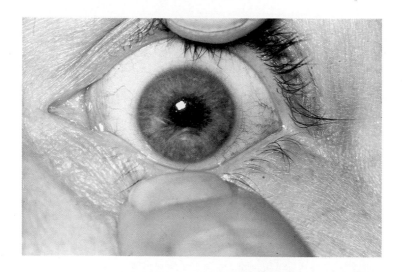

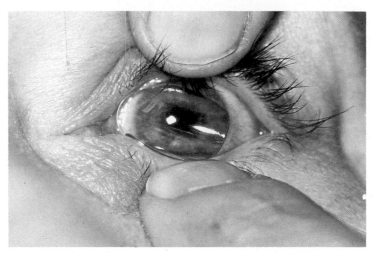

Fig. 26 Removal of a soft contact lens

However lens preservative intolerance develops in only a few cases, and usually after at least 6 months' use. So on neither count need this advice be taken too seriously if the eye drops *must* be used and the patient insists on wearing the lens.

It is of greater concern that a contact lens is not worn when there is an eye disorder, such as keratitis or conjunctivitis, in which the lens might be implicated. 'When in doubt, take it out' is sound advice for any contact lens wearer.

12

Squint and nystagmus

SQUINT

A squint is present when the image of an object falls on the fovea of one eye but not of the other.

CLASSIFICATION

a. Non-paralytic or concomitant.
b. Paralytic.

Non-paralytic squint

The development of binocular vision

The central part of the retina, the macula, is the only part with which detail can be seen, and an inborn reflex normally brings the image on to the macula. If an object is seen by both eyes, a reflex aligns the eyes to avoid diplopia. If some obstacle makes the binocular use of the eyes difficult, the child may suppress the image seen by one eye and concentrate on the other. Suppression leads to one eye squinting and, more importantly, to the development of amblyopia — 'lazy eye'. If amblyopia persists beyond the age of about 7 years it will be irreversible, with permanent loss of useful vision.

The main causes of squint in childhood are:

— Heredity.
— High degrees of refractive error.
— Ocular disease, preventing the proper development of vision.

Errors of refraction and squint

To look at a close object, it is necessary not only to focus the eyes by the use of accommodation but also to exercise convergence.

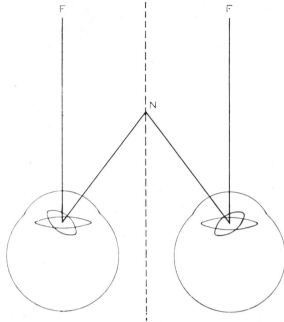

Fig. 27 The Accommodation–Convergence Relationship. If the eyes are considered, in the first instance, as regarding a distant object (F) a clear retinal image is obtained in each eye without any effort of either accommodation or convergence. On looking at a near object (N) a balanced relationship normally exists between the degree of accommodation exerted and the angle of convergence. In hypermetropia this relationship is upset.

In hypermetropia, if the amount of accommodation is out of proportion to the amount of convergence needed at a given distance (Fig. 27), the child may not be able to dissociate these functions, with resultant over-convergence.

Ocular disease and squint

If any ocular disorder prevents the proper development of binocular vision, a squint may result. Among possible causes are corneal opacities, cataract, retinal disease and optic atrophy.

Clinical varieties of concomitant squint:

— Convergent or divergent
— Constant or intermittent
— Uniocular or alternating

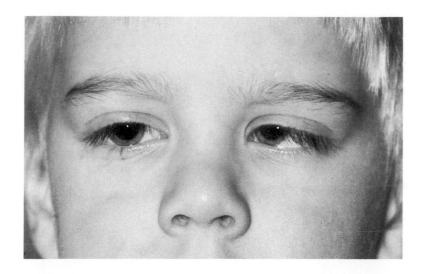

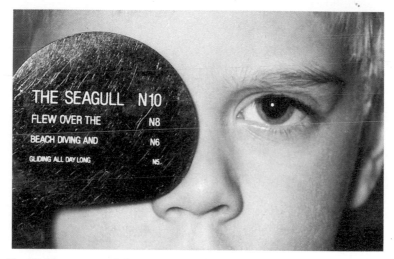

THE SEAGULL N10
FLEW OVER THE N8
BEACH DIVING AND N6
GLIDING ALL DAY LONG N5

Fig. 28 The cover test: left convergent squint

Presentation

Although it may be present from birth, onset is typically between 3 and 6 years. The squint, intermittent at first, is often noticed by someone other than the parents. It is usually more obvious when the child is tired, angry or unwell. A child does not 'grow out of' a squint and time spent waiting for spontaneous cure is wasted. If a child is only using one eye and is neglecting the other, the vision in the disused eye falls and this amblyopia can become permanent and irrecoverable.

Diagnosis

The commonest cause of a mistaken diagnosis is epicanthus, making the cornea seem closer to the midline that it actually is.

In any doubt, the relative positions of the bright reflexes from the cornea must be assessed. If the eyes are 'straight' the bright reflection of a torch will be symmetrical in the two eyes.

The other invaluable test is the *cover test* (Fig. 28). Ensuring that the child's attention is attracted, the eyes are covered in turn. If each eye remains stationary when its fellow eye is covered, no squint is present. If, however, on covering one eye, the opposite eye moves to take up fixation, this eye was originally squinting.

Treatment

The treatment of squint consists of the following steps, the detailed application of which will be decided by the ophthalmologist:

a. *Refraction*, providing spectacles if indicated (Fig. 29), and fundus examination.

b. *Occlusion of the fixing eye*, to force the amblyopic eye into activity.

c. *Orthoptic supervision*, to assess the state of binocular vision and to assist in the planning of surgery.

d. *Operation* may be required in the treatment of those who do not respond to the provision of glasses together with orthoptic treatment. Surgery is the only possible treatment in neglected cases showing incurable amblyopia, when the problem is purely cosmetic. General anaesthesia is necessary, but the hospital stay is short, the child going home as soon as he has fully recovered from the anaesthetic.

Divergent squint

This condition is much less common than convergent squint. It presents at a later age, is usually seen on distant gaze and is more obvious in bright light.

Treatment is surgical and the prognosis good.

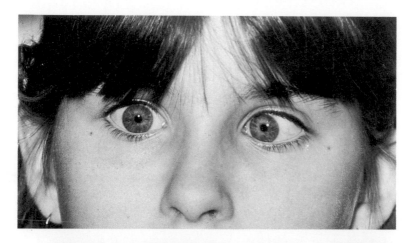

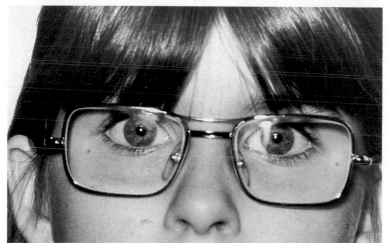

Fig. 29 Accommodative convergent squint, controlled in glasses

Paralytic squint

Usually seen in later life, these squints may be due to trauma, intracranial vascular accidents, aneurysms, and tumours.

Symptoms

The only symptom is diplopia, often leading to giddiness and nausea, and usually worse in one direction of the gaze.

Diagnosis

A marked squint may be obvious, or there may be limitation of movement of an eye.

The cause usually lies within the central nervous system; most paralytic squints occurring in the elderly are due to small arteriosclerotic lesions. Recovery usually takes place in a few weeks. A prism attached temporarily to the glasses is often helpful.

If recovery fails to occur and the patient remains incapacitated by diplopia, surgery will usually restore binocular vision, at least in the lower field of vision where problems with reading, coping with steps, and so on, are likely to arise.

A paralytic squint in an arteriosclerotic patient should be regarded as a minor stroke and may be the forerunner of a major cerebrovascular accident.

NYSTAGMUS

Nystagmus — involuntary, oscillatory movement of the eyes — is either jerky, with fast and slow components, or pendular. The cause may be in the labyrinthine or visual systems.

Jerky nystagmus is seen under certain circumstances in normal individuals. Examples in the vestibular system are the induction of nystagmus on caloric stimulation of the ears and on rotation of the head. In the visual system, optokinetic nystagmus occurs when objects are fixated in rapid succession, as when looking through the window of a moving train, and in 'end point' nystagmus the eyes oscillate on extreme lateral gaze.

Vestibular nystagmus occurs in disorders of the middle ear and its central connections, and of the cerebellum. The movements are jerky, with the fast component towards the side of the lesion.

Pendular nystagmus is seen in children whose vision is markedly impaired in both eyes at birth, or becomes so during the first year or two of life. It arises because the normal fixation reflexes cannot become established.

Congenital nystagmus is a fairly common inherited condition. The movements may be horizontal, vertical or rotatory. Usually there is one position of gaze in which they are at least marked, and the patient may adopt a compensatory head posture so that the eyes assume this position, thereby obtaining optimum vision. Corrective surgery or prisms sometimes help.

In the absence of other ocular disorders, most children with congenital nystagmus achieve good near vision, so they can read small print and cope with normal schooling. But their distance visual acuity is generally not better than 6/18 (Snellen). Hence parents should be warned that their child may not have good enough vision to be eligible for a driving licence (Ch. 16). This may have important consequences for employment.

Latent nystagmus is not apparent when both eyes are fixing but becomes manifest when either is covered. The condition is of no importance clinically unless the sight in one eye is unfortunately lost; but it may be the cause of failure at a sight test when each eye is tested separately. When tested with both eyes in use, vision is normal.

AMBLYOPIA (LAZY EYE)

Defined as reduced acuity in an eye without detectable disorder of the retina or visual pathways, amblyopia due to *squint* has been considered on p. 103. Other causes are *stimulus deprivation*, as in ptosis or congenital cataract, in which the defect must be corrected as early as possible if useful vision is to be achieved, and unequal refractive errors in the two eyes (*anisometropia*).

A difference in hypermetropia greater than 1 dioptre or in myopia greater than 3 dioptres may lead to amblyopia in the absence of a squint. Provided the refractive difference is not excessive, optical correction combined with occlusion of the eye with normal vision usually gives markedly improved, if not normal, acuity in the amblyopic eye. Best results are obtained under 6 or 7 years of age, but limited improvement may be obtained in older children. Inadequately corrected astigmatism may lead to partial amblyopia in both eyes.

Slight amblyopia, with reduced acuity when measured by reading Snellen test type lines, may escape detection with single letter-matching tests like the Sheridan Gardiner (p. 3). This phenomenon is known as 'crowding' and should be borne in mind when interpreting the results of letter-matching tests.

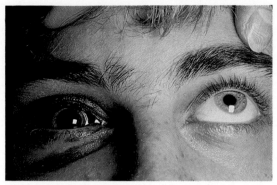

Plate 32 Blow-out fracture of orbit

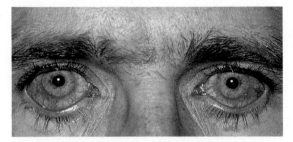

Plate 33 Conjunctivitis due to contact lens soaking solution

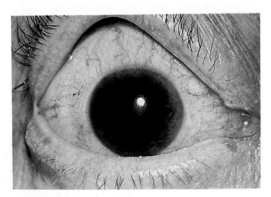

Plate 34 Acute angle-closure glaucoma

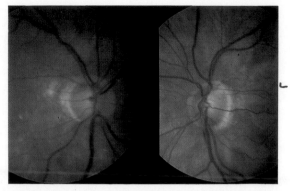

Plate 35 Optic discs in open-angle glaucoma. 75-year-old man, newly diagnosed. Right eye: thinning of neuro-retinal rim inferiorly, giving vertically oval cup; superior field loss. Left eye: splinter haemorrhage at lower disc margin; field almost intact. Intra-ocular pressures: right eye 31 mmHg, left 25 mmHg.

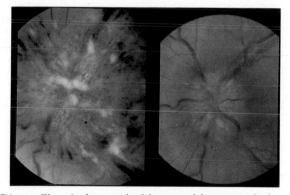

Plate 36 Disc swelling. 1: due to raised intra-cranial pressure. 2: due to optic neuritis

13

Glaucoma

Any condition in which intra-ocular pressure is higher than normal, with resulting damage to vision, may be defined as glaucoma. 21 mmHg is usually considered to be the upper normal limit. The balance between aqueous humour production and drainage determines intra-ocular pressure.

Aqueous is produced by the *ciliary body* and passes through the pupil to the anterior chamber, from which it drains in the *angle* formed by the anterior surface of the iris and the cornea.

Aqueous leaves the anterior chamber through pores in the trabecular meshwork, entering the *Canal of Schlemm*, an encircling channel at the corneo-scleral junction, and passes into the blood stream via the episcleral plexus of veins.

Glaucoma is classified according to the cause of the raised intra-ocular pressure: there are primary and secondary glaucomas (Table 11).

Table 11 Classification of glaucoma

Primary glaucoma	Secondary glaucoma
Congenital	Post-traumatic
Primary angle-closure	Uveitis
Primary open angle	Lens-induced
	Thrombotic
	Steroids
	(Others)

CONGENITAL GLAUCOMA (Buphthalmos)

Occasionally present at birth, this condition is so rare that a general practitioner is unlikely ever to see it; however early recognition is essential for successful treatment. Congenital abnormalities in the trabecular meshwork impede the drainage of aqueous.

The infant's eyes water profusely and are red and painful. The child is irritable and rubs its eyes. Attacks of pain may be intermittent in the early stages. The cornea has a ground glass appearance and becomes enlarged beyond the normal diameter of 10.5 mm. There may be splits in the deep layer of the cornea. The globe enlarges and the disc becomes cupped.

Any suspected case must be referred urgently. Treatment is surgical.

PRIMARY ANGLE-CLOSURE GLAUCOMA (Acute, congestive glaucoma)

Acute glaucoma is one of the emergencies in ophthalmology; it is rare below the age of 60. A general practitioner is unlikely to see more than one acute case in his lifetime.

Pathogenesis

Gradual shallowing of the anterior chamber as the lens enlarges with increasing age predisposes to angle closure glaucoma: it cannot develop in eyes with deep anterior chambers (Fig. 30). The intra-ocular pressure rises — usually suddenly. The pupil becomes fixed in mid-dilatation and, with increasing pressure, corneal oedema occurs.

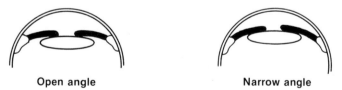

Open angle   Narrow angle

Fig. 30 Diagram of open and narrow angles

Angle-closure glaucoma may also develop gradually, with progressive closure of the drainage angle. Such cases are differentiated from open angle glaucoma by detailed examination of the angle with a special contact lens (gonioscope).

Presentation

Typically, the patient complains of sudden onset of pain with blurred vision (usually down to 'counting fingers' or 'hand movements'). One eye is affected, but the stress resulting from the attack may precipitate a similar situation in the other eye. Collapse and vomiting may occur if the pain is severe.

The eye is red, with corneal oedema preventing a clear view of the iris detail and the pupil is fixed and semi-dilated (Plate 34). Raised intra-ocular pressure is obvious on palpation of the closed eye through the upper lid: the eye feels stony hard.

The patient may give a previous history of visual disturbance, particularly seeing coloured haloes around white lights in the evening, perhaps with pain and blurring. These attacks may initially be self-limiting and relieved by sleep, during which the normal pupil constricts. Such a history requires referral as a glaucoma suspect, even without evidence of established angle closure.

The use of mydriatic drops to dilate the pupils for examination of the fundus — for example in the routine review of diabetics — may, very rarely, precipitate an attack of angle closure. In eyes seen to have shallow anterior chambers, demonstrable by shining a light obliquely on to the cornea and finding only part of the convex iris illuminated, these drops should be used with caution.

Management

All cases must be referred as emergencies. Hospital treatment is with intensive pilocarpine drops — usually 4%, instilled every minute for 5 minutes, and every 5 minutes for half an hour — and intravenous acetazolamide (Diamox) 500 mg. Additional medical treatment may be necessary and 2% pilocarpine is used prophylactically in the fellow eye. Definitive treatment is surgical — making a hole in the peripheral iris to permit the passage of aqueous into the anterior chamber, by-passing the pupil. This may be achieved either by peripheral iridectomy or laser iridotomy. Provided permanent damage has not occurred in the drainage angle by adhesion formation, the patient is then cured. The fellow eye usually requires prophylactic iridectomy or laser iridotomy.

PRIMARY OPEN-ANGLE GLAUCOMA (Chronic simple glaucoma)

A common and still incompletely understood condition, open-angle glaucoma occurs in about 2% of people over age 40 with increasing incidence in older age groups. It is bilateral and a common cause of blindness: early diagnosis gives the best chance of satisfactory treatment. Family history is of great importance — the incidence in first degree relatives of glaucoma sufferers is several times higher than in the general population. Siblings and children of patients with glaucoma are thus particularly at risk.

Pathogenesis

Drainage of aqueous at the trabecular meshwork is impeded, despite free access to the angle, for reasons that are not clear. The consequence is raised intra-ocular pressure which results in damage to the blood supply of the disc. This leads to characteristic atrophy of nerve fibres at the optic disc (cupping) (Fig. 31) and visual field defects which, if the pressure is not controlled, tend to progress to blindness.

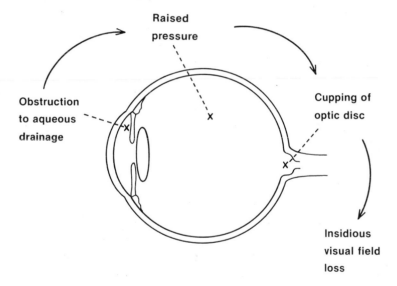

Fig. 31 Open-angle glaucoma (diagram)

It is common to find raised intra-ocular pressure without disc changes or field loss — termed 'ocular hypertension'. In these eyes it is assumed that the disc circulation, of which the most vulnerable part is the superficial vessel system supplied from the choroid, is adequate to maintain normal nutrition of the disc in spite of the adverse influence of raised intra-ocular pressure.

Steroid eye preparations cause raised intra-ocular pressure in susceptible individuals if they are used for more than a few weeks. Pressure checks are therefore mandatory. If increased pressure is found and the continued use of steroid considered essential, the ophthalmologist may decide to use one of the available steroids which are less prone to this side effect — fluoromethalone (FML) or clobetasone (Eumovate).

Risk factors in open-angle glaucoma, apart from increasing with age over 40 and with a family history, have been identified as high myopia, diabetes, ischaemic heart disease and a history of a bleeding episode requiring blood transfusion.

Diagnosis

Most cases are initially detected in the course of routine sight tests. Several surveys in the United Kingdom have shown that general practitioners had suspected the diagnosis in about 5% of patients referred to eye clinics and found to have glaucoma. The factors taken into account in making the diagnosis are:

— Cupping of the disc.
— Raised intra-ocular pressure.
— Visual field loss.

Cupping of the disc

This is the feature most accessible to the general practitioner and every opportunity should be taken to practise the assessment of discs for possible glaucomatous changes. All doubtful cases, as well as those with apparently obvious changes, should be referred for further assessment. In this way the general practitioners' share of the glaucoma referrals will increase! But it is not easy; even experts find it impossible to distinguish normal from glaucomatous discs with certainty.

The feature to look for particularly is the uniformity of width of the disc margin and symmetry in both eyes. Note should also be taken of:

1. *The size of the cup,* expressed as cup–disc ratio. 1.0 indicates complete cupping and 0.5 that the cup extends for half the overall disc diameter. 'Physiological' cupping is seen in healthy eyes, but a high cup–disc ratio carries a strong suspicion of glaucoma.

2. *A vertically oval cup* (vertical cup–disc ratio greater than horizontal) usually correlates with glaucomatous field loss (Plate 35).

3. *Asymmetry* between the disc cupping in the two eyes frequently suggests glaucoma.

4 *Haemorrhage* at the disc margin, suggesting circulatory embarrassment in the optic nerve-head, makes a diagnosis of glaucoma likely (Plate 35).

5. *Pallor* of the disc is more difficult to evaluate: it may be of significance, but cupping is a more reliable sign. Advanced cases of glaucoma always have pale discs.

Fundus examination showing extensive retinal haemorrhages due to retinal vein occlusion (p. 74) indicates immediate referral. A venous occlusion may be the presenting feature of glaucoma.

Raised intra-ocular pressure

There are as many pitfalls in intra-ocular pressure measurement and the conclusions drawn from it as from disc assessment. Guessing the pressure by palpation of globe is useless, except in the extreme

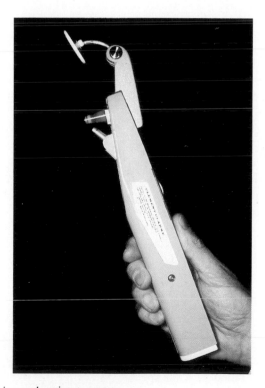

Fig. 32 Perkins applanation tonometer

case of acute angle-closure glaucoma (p. 113). It is by no means incumbent on general practitioners to measure intra-ocular pressure (tonometry), but if a doctor decides to do so it is probably most satisfactory to obtain a hand held applanation tonometer (Fig. 32) and practise regularly to become proficient. The increasing incidence of open angle glaucoma over age 40 makes tonometry a valuable screening procedure in routine medical checks, though usually outside the scope of general practice.

Routine tonometry is usually carried out in the course of eye examination for refraction: most people over age 45 use reading glasses and have periodic tests thereafter. Patients found at refraction to have intra-ocular pressures over 21 mmHg are commonly referred to the general practitioner. It helps the ophthalmologist considerably if the referral letter is accompanied by all the details given on the report, as well as any other medical details the general practitioner may consider relevant.

Visual field examination

To detect glaucomatous loss at an early stage is time-consuming and may require complex apparatus. This aspect of diagnosis is therefore outside the scope of general practice.

Once field loss is sufficiently advanced to attract the patient's attention, the glaucoma is likely to be far advanced. Early diagnosis is the key to successful management.

Glaucomatous field loss tends to be more severe in patients with generalised arteriosclerosis, due probably to poor perfusion of the optic nerve head. Sudden exacerbation of field loss may be seen after acute illnesses such as coronary thrombosis, severe gastrointestinal haemorrhage or major surgery in which there has been a period of significantly lowered blood pressure.

Field loss and disc cupping without raised intra-ocular pressure represent failure of the disc circulation without impaired drainage of aqueous. This condition is termed 'low-tension glaucoma'. Treatment is difficult.

Management

All cases of suspected glaucoma should be referred. Priority should be indicated. It is preferable that treatment be withheld until after the first consultation with the specialist in order that a true base-line assessment can be made.

Raised pressure alone, without disc or field changes ('ocular hypertension') requires specialist follow-up but is not usually treated. If there is any evidence of change in the disc appearance or visual field loss, treatment for glaucoma must be given.

The choice is between drug therapy by eye drops (or, rarely, oral agents), conventional glaucoma drainage surgery and laser trabeculoplasty. It is usual to try drug therapy with drops initially. The other means are reserved for those who do not respond satisfactorily, due either to failure to tolerate the regime or its ineffectiveness, manifested by persistently raised pressure and progressive field loss. However a growing body of ophthalmic opinion favours immediate laser trabeculoplasty or surgical trabeculectomy.

Medical

The drugs commonly used and their side effects are listed in Table 12. Most frequently prescribed are timolol (Timoptol) 0.25% or 0.5% and pilocarpine 0.5% to 4%, sometimes combined with a wetting agent. Pilocarpine is also available as slow-release 'Ocuserts' which are inserted into the lower conjunctival fornix and changed weekly.

Patient 'compliance' is all-important, and it is the responsibility of the ophthalmologist, supported by the general practitioner, to ensure that the patient understands why glaucoma drugs have been prescribed and that their aim is the preservation of useful sight, rather than the improvement of vision.

The general practitioner must be aware of the potentially dangerous side effects of timolol (Table 12). If in doubt, stop the drug and refer.

Surgical

Patients in whom glaucoma is not adequately controlled by medical treatment require surgery to bring the pressure to 21 mmHg or less and prevent further field loss. The surgical procedure most commonly used is trabeculectomy, in which a small block of tissue is removed from the trabecular meshwork. A drainage 'bleb' or blister usually results and can be seen behind the limbus under the upper lid.

Surgical treatment may need to be supplemented post-operatively by drops. The operation may be done under general or local anaesthesia. Accelerated cataract formation is a major disadvantage of glaucoma surgery.

Table 12　Drugs commonly used in open-angle glaucoma

Group	Name	'Trade' name	Inconvenient side effects	Serious side effects
Miotics	Pilocarpine (0.5%–4%) up to 4 × daily	Isopto-carpine SNO-Pilo Ocuserts	Brow ache Small pupil Transient myopia	
	Ecothiopate (0.03%–1.2%) twice daily	Phospholine iodide	Brow ache Small pupil Transient myopia	Iris cysts Cataract Pseudo-cholinesterase depletion (succinyl choline apnoea risk)
Sympathomimetics	Adrenaline (1%) twice daily	Eppy, Simplene	Red eyes Local irritation Tachycardia	Angle closure with narrow angles
	Dipivefrin hydrochloride (0.1%) twice daily	Propine		
* Adrenergic antagonists	Timolol maleate (0.25–0.5%) twice daily	Timoptol Timoptic	Local irritation Skin rash	Exacerbation of obstructive airways disease. Dangerous in heart block and cardiac failure
Combined preparation	Guanethidine and adrenaline (1 + 0.2% to 5 + 1%) twice daily	Ganda	Red eyes Local irritation Headache Tachycardia Ptosis	Angle closure with narrow angles
Carbonic Anhydrase inhibitors	Acetazolamide 0.5 g to 1 g daily	Diamox Diamox 'sustets'	Paraesthesiae Gastrointestinal disturbance	Urinary calculi Agranulocytosis Gastrointestinal ulceration Weight loss
	Dichlorphenamide 100–200 mg daily	Daranide Oratrol		Electrolyte imbalance

*other drugs in this group, e.g. Teoptic and Betoptic, are now available.

An alternative and increasingly popular treatment is *laser trabeculoplasty*. About 100 small burns are applied with an argon laser to the trabecular meshwork. This is an out-patient procedure without significant complications. It appears to be successful in many cases, but its long-term efficacy awaits firm evaluation.

Treatment by conventional drainage surgery or laser trabeculoplasty may free patients from the need to take regular medication, but most are advised to have periodic checks to ensure that the glaucoma remains satisfactorily controlled.

Glaucoma requires a life-time of regular ophthalmic supervision and the general practitioner may be asked to make inquiries of defaulters. He also has a role in advising relatives of glaucoma patients, who may be at risk, to seek appropriate examination.

SECONDARY GLAUCOMA

Uveitis

Iritis or iridocyclitis may be accompanied by raised intra-ocular pressure, usually settling as the inflammation subsides. Drugs to reduce intra-ocular pressure may be needed in addition to those prescribed to control the uveitis (see p. 58).

Lens-induced glaucoma

A hypermature cataract, seen as a white opacity in the pupil, may degenerate and obstruct aqueous drainage by the collection of material in the trabeculum, or swell and cause angle-closure glaucoma. Any patient with a red painful eye and a dense, mature cataract should be referred urgently.

Post-traumatic glaucoma

Blunt injury, usually causing hyphaema (p. 57) originally, may predispose to glaucoma by damaging the drainage angle. This accounts for a number of unilateral cases of open-angle glaucoma. Patients who have sustained significant injury to an eye should be watched with more than usual vigilance for open-angle glaucoma and should report the history of injury when undergoing routine eye tests.

Thrombotic glaucoma

Associated with rubeosis iridis (common causes: proliferative diabetic retinopathy and central retinal vein occlusion with ischaemia), this presents as pain in a blind eye, (see p. 75, 81). New vessels are visible on the surface of the iris. Treatment is unsatisfactory.

Drugs

The use of steroid drops or ointment in or around the eye for periods longer than a week or two leads to raised intra-ocular pressure in susceptible individuals. Two topical steroid preparations are available which show this effect to a lesser degree — fluoromethalone (FML) and clobetasone (Eumovate).

14

The visual pathway

OPTIC NERVE

The general practitioner can inspect the optic nerve at the optic disc, and assess its function by testing pupil reactions (p. 7), visual acuity, colour recognition and visual fields. Complex equipment is needed to test function electrically.

Disorders of the optic nerve producing pallor of the optic disc (optic atrophy) are listed in Table 13.

Table 13   Causes of optic atrophy

Trauma
Ischaemia — giant cell arteritis and arteriosclerosis
Optic neuritis
Compressive lesions of the visual pathway
Toxic or nutritional optic nerve damage
Glaucoma
Retinitis pigmentosa
Resolved papilloedema

1. *Trauma*. Usually a severe blow to the eye or side of the head. Apart from loss of vision, the only sign may be an afferent pupillary defect. Skull X-rays are advisable, but may show no fracture. Optic atrophy develops in 6–8 weeks.

2. *Ischaemic optic neuropathy* has two common causes:

a. *Giant cell arteritis*. A medical emergency usually occurring over age 60. There may be prodromal symptoms of temporal arteritis — malaise, weight loss, pain on chewing, discomfort wearing a hat and headache. Sudden and profound loss of vision occurs and a pale, swollen disc is seen with loss of direct pupillary reaction. Episodes of transient visual loss (amaurosis fugax) may occur first.

123

The diagnosis is all but confirmed by finding a significantly raised ESR (usually over 50 mm/hr) or plasma viscosity (usually over 1.9). Immediate treatment with high dosage steroid by mouth is essential: the usual starting dose is prednisolone 120 mg daily, reducing as the ESR falls.

The patient may be referred for a temporal artery biopsy, but treatment must come first. Failure to start early and adequate steroid therapy may result in the even more disastrous loss of vision in the second eye.

b. *Arteriosclerotic ischaemic optic neuropathy* presents similarly, but may be seen in younger patients. There is no associated arteritis — the ESR is normal. Visual loss may be less profound and its onset more gradual. The optic disc is swollen.

Management. Having excluded giant cell arteritis, other factors predisposing to arterial occlusion should be sought — hypertension, diabetes and lipid disorders. There is less risk of bilateral involvement than in giant cell arteritis.

3. *Optic neuritis.* Termed 'retrobulbar' neuritis if the swelling is sufficiently near the optic nerve head to cause disc swelling, the onset is usually in the 20–45 age group, but children may be affected. The cause, like that of disseminated sclerosis, is not known. There is a positive association with histocompatibility antigen HLA-DR2.

The patient complains of impaired vision — maybe as poor as mere perception of light, impaired colour discrimination (best shown with a red target) and a central visual field defect. The eye may be tender to touch, with discomfort on looking to the side. The afferent pupillary defect is, in mild cases, an oscillating response to direct light. The swinging light test (p. 7) demonstrates impaired function in the affected optic nerve.

Treatment does not affect the outcome of optic neuritis though ACTH or steroids may be recommended to speed recovery of vision. Most patients regain normal or near-normal vision after the first episode. More than 50% of previously healthy patients developing optic neuritis are found on long-term follow-up to develop other symptoms of demyelinating disease. The exact proportion developing disseminated sclerosis is uncertain, but some undoubtedly have no further neurological illness.

Certain drugs, particularly ethambutol, may cause optic neuritis.

4. *Compressive lesions of the optic nerve* are considered on page 126. Any patient with temporal visual field loss or unexplained loss

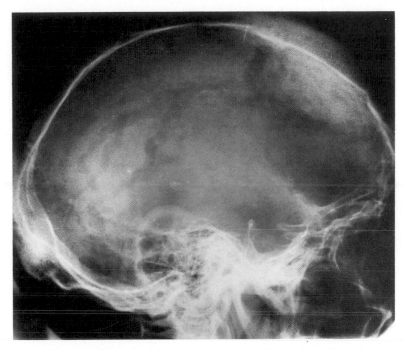

Fig. 33 Lateral radiograph of skull showing pituitary fossa enlarged by tumour. Note sloping, 'double' floor of fossa and erosion of posterior clinoids

of vision should raise suspicion of a pituitary tumour or other compressive lesion. The highest-yielding investigation is lateral X-ray of the pituitary fossa (Fig. 33). Computerized tomography (CT) scanning is more informative.

5. *Tobacco/alcohol optic neuropathy.* Older people who smoke, drink heavily and eat poorly are most at risk. Pipe smokers are predominant.

Presentation is with gradually decreasing visual acuity. Defective colour perception and a characteristic central visual field defect can be demonstrated. Both eyes are affected.

Treatment is by stopping smoking, withdrawing alcohol and giving multivitamins by mouth and hydroxycobalamine (Neo-cytamen) by injection: 1000 μg daily for a week, weekly for a month and 3-monthly thereafter. The response to treatment is good.

6. *Glaucoma* — see page 115.

7. *Retinitis pigmentosa* — see page 86.

PAPILLOEDEMA (Plate 36).

Swelling of the optic disc may be due to papilloedema or pseudo-papilloedema. The distinction may not be easy; all cases of doubt should be referred immediately.

Signs of papilloedema:

Disc swelling
Haemorrhages near disc
Loss of central optic cup
Lack of pulsation of central retinal vein
Dilatation of retinal veins
Central visual acuity usually preserved

Papilloedema may be due to:

1. Raised intracranial pressure: usually with headaches, worse in the morning, and on straining. Vomiting and localising signs may occur.
2. Ischaemic optic neuropathy (p. 123).
3. Malignant hypertension (p. 72).
4. Optic neuritis (p. 124).

INTERFERENCE WITH THE VISUAL PATHWAY

The eye may serve as a guide to the presence and location of intracranial disease by the finding of visual field changes: rough testing can be carried out by the confrontation method (p. 3).

Although the lesions producing visual field defects are multiple, the types of visual loss that they cause are characteristic (p. 128).

If the lesion is *in front of the optic chiasma*, the defect is strictly uniocular with an afferent pupillary defect demonstrable by the swinging light test (p. 7). The optic disc is pale and atrophic.

Lesions *at the optic chiasma* produce bitemporal hemianopia, due to interference with the crossing fibres which carry impulses from the nasal half of each retina. This is typical of pituitary tumours and the loss of field is generally asymmetrical. Impaired colour recognition is an early sign.

Behind the chiasma any interference with the visual pathway (Fig. 34) will affect both eyes.

The right optic tract, optic radiation and visual cortex receive impulses from the right halves of both retinae and damage here is projected into the left visual field. Similarly, the right visual field is served by the left visual pathway.

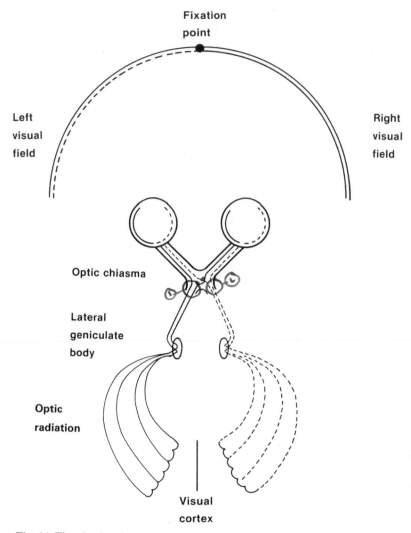

Fig. 34 The visual pathway

A lesion behind the chiasma, therefore, leads to a homonymous field defect: lying in the same half of the field of vision of both eyes.

Running through the brain to terminate in the visual cortex at the occipital pole, the fibres of the visual pathway follow a consistent and well-defined pattern. Knowledge of the distribution of these fibres, combined with detailed analysis of visual field defects, allows accurate localisation of a lesion.

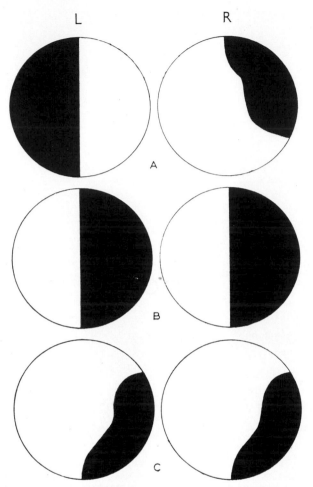

Fig. 35 Visual field changes, charted as seen by the patient. (A) Bitemporal hemianopia. Pituitary lesion. Complete in the left eye. Incomplete in right. (B) Homonymous hemianopia. Complete lesion of left visual pathway. Right-sided hemianopia. (C) Incomplete homonymous hemianopia

Examples of typical visual field defects are given in Figure 35.

The results of field defect analysis together with the CT scan are invaluable in the investigation of intracranial disease.

By far the commonest cause of homonymous field loss is a stroke involving an optic radiation. This defect can be readily demonstrated by the general practitioner using the technique described on page 5.

MOTOR AND SENSORY LESIONS

As well as producing visual field defects, intracranial lesions may interfere with ocular movements and produce sensory changes.

Disorders of the pupil

The technique for testing pupil reactions is described on page 7.

The following are some of the commoner pupillary abnormalities:

Tonic, or Holmes-Adie, pupil. The tonic pupil is semi-dilated and at first seems unreactive to light. If, however, the patient is exposed to bright light for some minutes, the pupil contracts slowly and dilates equally slowly on return to the dark.

This occurs unilaterally in young people and is often associated with absence of the deep tendon reflexes in the lower limbs. The condition is not associated with serious neurological disease.

Optic (retrobulbar) neuritis (see p. 124)

Horner's syndrome. The complete Horner's syndrome comprises a small pupil, ptosis, diminished sweating on the affected side of the face, and apparent enophthalmos. The condition is sometimes congenital but, if due to an active process, is caused by disease or injury affecting the sympathetic pathways (see Fig. 11, p. 22).

The blind eye. In complete lesions of the optic nerve, as after injury, perception of light is lost and with it the direct reaction of the pupil to light (afferent pupillary defect).

Accidental mydriasis. A common cause of dilatation of the pupil without other signs is accidental exposure to mydriatic drugs. This may be due to the use of eye drops or ointment ordered for another patient, or to contamination of the fingers and inadvertent transfer of the drug to the eye.

15

The orbit

Orbital disease usually presents as *proptosis* because the rigid walls of the orbit only permit expansion of contents anteriorly. Proptosis can be most easily seen when standing behind the seated patient. Measurement is carried out from the side, holding a ruler against the bony edge of the lateral wall of the orbit and estimating its distance from the apex of the cornea in profile. The two sides can be compared.

Double vision and displacement of the globe are also evidence of orbital disease.

Dysthyroid eye disease (Fig. 36)

The commonest orbital problem — proptosis may be unilateral or bilateral. CT scanning is indicated if the diagnosis is in doubt.

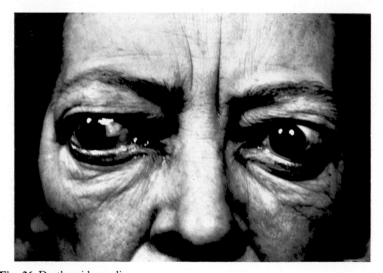

Fig. 36 Dysthyroid eye disease

Other signs are:

1. *Lid retraction* — the superior corneal margin is visible: under normal circumstances the lid covers the upper third of the cornea.

2. *Lid lag* — the upper lid lags behind the eye in vertical movements.

3. *Double vision* — may result from involvement and tethering of the extra-ocular muscles.

The underlying cause of dysthyroid eye disease is not clear, but it may occur at any stage in the course of thyrotoxicosis and its treatment. Patients should be referred for ophthalmic assessment if complications prove a cosmetic embarrassment or a risk to sight. Hypothyroidism during the treatment of thyrotoxicosis may exacerbate eye complications and should be avoided.

Ophthalmic complications

1. Double vision.
2. Exposure keratitis (see p. 54).
3. Retinal or optic nerve circulatory impairment and secondary glaucoma.

Threat to vision may necessitate treatment with high doses of steroid (120 mg prednisolone daily) or immuno-suppressive drugs (more than half the patients respond). Surgical decompression of the orbit is rarely needed.

Dysthyroid eye disease is self-limiting. Most cases return to nearly normal appearance eventually. The condition may persist for several years.

Orbital cellulitis

Infection of the orbital contents leads to painful proptosis, difficulty opening the eye, and redness of the skin. There is usually purulent discharge.

The commonest *cause* is sinus infection, usually ethmoiditis, confirmed by X-ray. Skin infections, injuries and metastatic infection may occasionally cause orbital cellulitis.

Management should be in hospital. Drainage of pus from the orbit or sinuses may be needed in addition to intensive antibiotic treatment.

Orbital tumours

Proptosis may be due to a tumour. If the displacement is axial, the tumour is likely to be within the cone of extra-ocular muscles. CT scanning is of great value in diagnosis.

Carotico-cavernous fistula

Causes proptosis with engorged collateral blood vessels and pulsation of the globe. An orbital bruit may be heard. The patients are elderly.

Trauma

Blunt injury of the orbit may cause a 'blow-out' fracture. There is enophthalmos, limitation of gaze (usually upwards), and diplopia (see p. 92).

16

Visual standards

Screening of children for visual defects

The details of assessments of vision in apparently healthy children vary, but the following is a typical screening policy:

at 6 weeks	screen for — congenital cataract (red reflex) — anatomical defects — squint — visual attention
at 8 months	screen for — fixation and following — squint (cover test)
at 3 years	screen for — squint (cover test) — visual acuity (Sheridan Gardiner test at 3 metres) — refer if 3/6 or worse in either eye
at school entry	screen for — squint (cover test) — visual acuity (Sheridan Gardiner test at 6 metres) — refer if 6/12 or less in either eye
during school	screen every other year with Snellen test type or other screening device (e.g. Keystone screener): check for colour vision defect at 10 years.

Some children of school age who are disinclined to read, and whose educational achievements are unsatisfactory, are hypermetropic. The degree of hypermetropia may be insufficient to impair distance acuity, so the child passes a routine vision check; but reading is an effort. Children with reading difficulty should be referred for refraction.

Most teachers and parents are nowadays aware of the possibility that a child with reading or writing difficulties may be dyslexic. Specialist advice is available from educational psychologists.

Occupational visual standards

The visual standards set for employment in the Services and in industry are complex. Advice may be obtained from the following United Kingdom sources, among others:

Army	Department of General Practice, Royal Army Medical College, Millbank, London (or local Recruiting Office)
British Airways	BA Medical Service, Heathrow, London
British Rail	Regional Medical Officer at regional HQ
Dept of Transport	Driver and Vehicle Licensing Directorate, Swansea (includes HGV and PSV)
Merchant Navy	General Council of British Shipping, Broomielaw, Glasgow (or local Board of Trade Examination Centre)
RAF	Local Recruiting Office
Royal Navy	Department of General Practice, Royal Naval Hospital, Haslar, Gosport (or local recruiting Office)

The principal visual criterion for employment is central visual acuity: colour vision is important in some jobs. There are variations between authorities as to whether the wearing of spectacles is permitted and, if so, of what strength.

The following are some of the main requirements:

Army

Most Regiments and Corps require corrected vision of 6/12 in each eye, or 6/6 right and 6/36 left.

British Airways

Pilots — corrected acuity of 6/9 in each eye. Spectacles allowed. Colour vision to Trade test.
Cabin Crew — 6/6, corrected, in each eye.
Ground Staff — standards depend on Grade.

British Rail

6/6 right and left on entry demanded of those who drive, or work on or near the track, with emphasis on the recognition of coloured signals. Spectacles allowed in later years. In lower categories, monocular vision may be acceptable.

Department of Transport

Motor-car drivers. Vision tested on recognition of number plates. 'Slightly better than 6/12' is the nearest Snellen equivalent. Monocular vision no bar.

'A driving licence may not be granted to a person who suffers from some other disability (including a disorder of the eye) which is likely to cause the driving of a vehicle by him to be a source of danger to the public.'

HGV and PSV. 6/9 in the better, and 6/12 in the worse eye, corrected. Any pathological visual field defect is a bar. A 1981 standard for uncorrected static visual acuity of 6/60 in either eye separately is required.

Significant loss of visual field in both eyes — for example, homonymous hemianopia or advanced glaucoma — bars any form of driving licence, even if satisfactory central acuity is achieved.

Merchant Navy

6/6–6/9 (glasses not allowed) for Deck Officers, and Ratings taking look-out duty. Colour vision to Trade test. Other Crew — 6/12 or less. Less good eye must be 6/60 or better.

RAF

Pilots — 6/12–6/12, corrected to 6/6–6/6. Good colour vision. Non-flying — Minimum standards: 6/60, 6/60, correcting to 6/9 in each eye. Exact requirements vary by trade.

Royal Navy

	Better eye		Worse eye
1.	6/9 N5	without glasses	6/12 N5
2.	6/12 N5	without glasses	6/12 N5
	6/6 N5	with glasses	6/6 N5
3.	6/6 N5	with or without glasses	6/24 N10
	6/9 N5		6/18 N10
	6/12 N5		6/12 N10

The higher standards are demanded for Seamen Officers and Fleet Air Arm Aircrew. Other entrants are graded according to the visual standards of the Branch.

17

Blindness and partial sight

The term 'blindness' does not necessarily imply total loss of sight. From the point of view of the Social Services, an individual is 'blind' when 'unable to perform any work for which eyesight is essential'. (Note — this definition does not mean 'unable to follow his previous occupation'.) In general, if the visual acuity is below 3/60 the above criterion is satisfied, though certain defects in the visual field may justify registration as 'blind' when the acuity is better than this.

Partial Sightedness, by definition, is a condition in which substantial and permanent handicap exists, short of that requiring registration as 'blind'. This usually implies vision within the range 3/60 to 6/60, but coincident defects such as severe visual field loss may allow registration in the presence of visual acuity better than 6/60.

Registers of the Blind and of the Partially Sighted are maintained by the Social Services Departments in each area in the U.K.

There follows a summary of the principal benefits available to those registered as handicapped on account of defective vision. The Social Work Department will provide assistance and advice, and it should be noted that some of the items listed are not available to the Partially Sighted, but only to the Blind.

— Reduction in cost of TV Licence.
— Some travel concessions.
— Postal concessions on articles for the Blind.
— Free Licence for Guide Dog.
— Increased Supplementary Benefit, if applicable.
— Blind Persons Income Tax relief.
— Rating relief on part or feature of house needed specifically on account of disability.
— Special Visual Aids, available through the Hospital Eye Service.
— Advice on household management.
— Education of visually handicapped children.

— Training in Braille and other reading methods.
— Hobbies and handicrafts.
— Aids, appliances and games.
— Braille controls for cookers, etc.
— Talking books and tape recorders.
— Large Print books, from local Libraries.
— Training and rehabilitation in Workshops for the Blind.

Some useful addresses in the United Kingdom:

— Royal National Institute for the Blind
224 Great Portland Street
London WIN 6AA

— Partially Sighted Society
Breaston
Derby DE7 3UE

— British Talking Book Service for the Blind
Nuffield Library
Mount Pleasant
Wembley
Middlesex

— British Wireless for the Blind Fund
(contact through Social Services Dept)

— Telephone for the Blind Fund
Mynthurst
Leigh
Nr Reigate
Surrey

Index

JOURNEY BEYOND
THE VILLAGE
WALLS AND INTO
DANGER.

◇▽◇▽◇▽◇▽◇▽◇▽◇

DISCOVER A NEW WORLD OF
INCREDIBLE MONSTERS.

◇▽◇▽◇▽◇▽◇▽◇▽◇

CAN LEO KEEP THE SECRET OF
THE GUARDIANS?

◇▽◇▽◇▽◇▽◇▽◇▽◇

WHERE WILL LEO'S MAP
TAKE HIM NEXT?

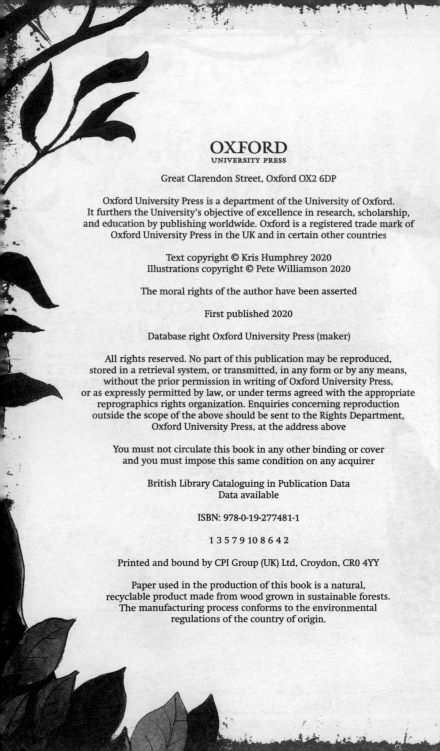

OXFORD
UNIVERSITY PRESS

Great Clarendon Street, Oxford OX2 6DP

Oxford University Press is a department of the University of Oxford.
It furthers the University's objective of excellence in research, scholarship,
and education by publishing worldwide. Oxford is a registered trade mark of
Oxford University Press in the UK and in certain other countries

British Library Cataloguing in Publication Data
Data available

ISBN: 978-0-19-277481-1

1 3 5 7 9 10 8 6 4 2

Printed and bound by CPI Group (UK) Ltd, Croydon, CR0 4YY

Paper used in the production of this book is a natural,
recyclable product made from wood grown in sustainable forests.
The manufacturing process conforms to the environmental
regulations of the country of origin.